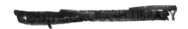
A Patient's PERSPECTIVE

Tips for Your Doctor Visits and More

Patricia Cyr

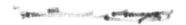

ISBN: 1463648804
ISBN 13: 9781463648800

Library of Congress Control Number: 2011911142
CreateSpace, North Charleston, SC

I dedicate this book to my husband, Dave, who has supported and loved me despite my chronic health conditions, to Rosemary for her genuine encouragement to those with interstitial cystitis, and to my family and friends who have listened endlessly to my journey as a patient.

Contents

Preface

This book helps you get the most out of visits with your doctors and other practitioners. It reveals common obstacles that you might encounter with your medical care and offers advice on how to deal with them effectively. May the tips I offer and experiences I share empower you. This book gives you emotional strength and encouragement to face the challenges that our health-care system presents.

I've lived with chronic illnesses for many years. My journey began in 1986 when I was diagnosed with interstitial cystitis, a chronic bladder condition. I later developed endometriosis, ovarian cancer, fibromyalgia, back problems, hypoglycemia, and Morton's neuromas. After each of my medical appointments, I kept notes about my experiences as a patient and services that could be improved. Over time, I realized that my notes were substantial enough to become a guide to share with others. I became an educated patient by asking medical professionals numerous questions and by listening to the medical experiences of other patients.

This book is not, in any manner, intended to be disrespectful to practitioners. Examples of my own experiences are given to provide insights into circumstances that other patients might face. I hope that not only patients but also practitioners will read this book. Practitioners will then gain a better understanding of what patients go through.

All practitioner names have been kept confidential. I have the utmost respect for doctors who do their best to restore patients to good health.

Acknowledgments

Special thanks to Gail Cocker, Dave Cyr, Patty Finch Dewey, Carra Leah Hood, and Kathy Ludlam for their technical and inspirational support with this book.

I also give thanks to Bobbie Christmas, Erin Cronin, and Elizabeth Tilley Hinkle, each of whom edited parts of this book.

I thank Martha Beth Lewis, PhD, for her grammatical advice.

I am deeply appreciative of patients who shared their medical journey with me and who realize that our medical system is in great need of change.

Disclaimer

Nothing in this book should be taken as the practice of medicine or law. This book is not intended as a substitute for the advice, treatment, or diagnosis by physicians or other practitioners. This book is not intended as a substitute for legal advice. The author is not, and does not profess to be, a doctor, dentist, lawyer, counselor, or medical professional. Consult a competent medical doctor regarding your own medical treatment and advice. If you are in need of legal advice, consult a competent attorney. If you are in need of counseling, seek a competent professional counselor, psychologist, or psychiatrist. The author disclaims all responsibility for any liability, injury, loss, or risk incurred as a consequence of reading and applying any content of this book.

The URLs displayed in this book refer to existing websites on the Internet at the time this book was written. Visitors to the websites displayed in this book should seek the advice of an appropriately qualified professional.

This book focuses on medical care in the United States of America.

❦❧❦❧

Appointment Issues

Making Appointments

Before you make an appointment, be confident that you have selected a good doctor.

If you need to see a physician, you can use several resources to find one. Family doctors can offer a wealth of information about specialists in the area. Nurses know a great deal about doctors' reputations. You can even ask nurses and doctors who they go to. They might not share that information, but it's worth asking. Ask your friends and other patients which doctors they prefer. Don't make a hasty conclusion based on just one or two comments from others. People vary in what characteristics and traits they value in a doctor. You can also contact patient advocacy groups to see if they can help you locate a good doctor. Many hospitals have measures to help you locate doctors. Ask librarians for online resources and magazines that list top-rated doctors in the United States and your local area.

Use care when selecting a family physician. It's best to have a family doctor who is both personable and competent. If you have confidence in your family doctor, you'll also feel confident about the specialists that he or she suggests. Good family doctors are important, because they are usually coordinators for patients' medical care.

If your insurance plan has in-network doctors and out-of-network doctors, check with your insurance carrier to see if the doctor you are considering is on its list as an in-network provider. Your costs will usually be less with an in-network provider. Some of my doctors are out-of-network, but I choose to see them anyway because I think their expertise is worth the extra cost.

When you select surgeons, consider which hospital(s) they perform surgeries at. Be sure the surgeons are associated with a reputable hospital. Check to see if the hospital is accredited by the Joint Commission, which is recognized nationwide as a symbol of quality.[1] They have numerous standards that a hospital must meet in order to be accredited by them.[2] You can reach them at 630-792-5000.

Some hospitals have more experience than others in treating particular medical conditions. It can benefit you to ask a hospital what diseases and treatments it specializes in. I would also walk into the hospital that you are considering and see if it looks clean and well-maintained. Call your insurance carrier and ask what type of coverage you have for a particular hospital.

After selecting local physicians, contact your state Department of Public Health and ask if the doctors are licensed to practice in your state. Also ask if there are complaints against those doctors. If your state Department of Public Health can't provide you with the information you need, it should be able to refer you to another agency that can help you. If the doctor you selected practices only in a state other than where you reside, contact that state's Department of Public Health.

Try to find out if the doctors you selected are board-certified, which ensures that they have passed certain exams within their area of specialization. It does not guarantee that they will be excellent doctors, but at least you know they have met reputable standards. You can sometimes find out if a doctor is board-certified by contacting the American Board of Medical Specialties.[3] You can reach them at 1-866-275-2267. If the customer service specialist can't find your doctor's name on its list, ask if the board has current information as of that day. Doctors that were recently certified may not appear on the list yet. If the representative still can't find the doctor's name, it's possible that the doctor wanted to keep such information private.[4]

If you know that a doctor previously practiced in another state, you can call that state's Board of Medical Examiners to be sure there were no complaints against the physician when he or she practiced there. If the Board of Medical Examiners doesn't have that information, it may be able to direct you to an appropriate agency that can assist you.

Some specialists will not see you unless another doctor referred you to them.

Don't base your decision to see a doctor solely on a rating.

There are websites that allow patients to rate their doctors and allow the public to view those ratings. Be careful how you interpret those types of ratings. What one patient views as a negative experience with a doctor, another might not. If, however, you see a multitude of negative or positive comments about a doctor's attitude, you should consider that. There may also be several patients who have had a good or poor experience with specific doctors, but never rated them. Unless a large percentage of patients provide ratings, I don't think too much weight can be put on the validity of the overall statistics.

I imagine that the issue of rating a doctor is controversial, and I believe it's still in somewhat of an infancy stage. I support a standardized system in which the majority of a physician's patients participate. I am not mentioning specific websites to view for ratings because I think better guidelines need to be established to enhance the credibility of such sites.

Ask the office what its procedure is for scheduling appointments.

The first time you make an appointment to see a physician, don't expect that there will be an opening soon. Sometimes an opening will be available within a few weeks. With many specialists, however, you may need to wait several months for an appointment. I've sometimes had to set up appointments four months in advance to see dermatologists and orthopedists. If there are few specialists in your geographic area, appointment slots could fill up quickly. There might be an especially long wait for a doctor who has a fabulous reputation. If you think you require more urgent attention, inform the doctor's office. They may be able to get you in sooner.

The process of scheduling follow-up appointments varies from office to office. Some places want you to schedule a year or more in advance. If you try to make appointments that far ahead in other offices, they may be surprised that you want to book so soon. When I tried booking several months in advance at one office, the staff expressed concern that I might cancel the appointment if my schedule changed. Also, some offices don't know too far in advance what days their doctors will be in the office.

Ask where the doctors practice.

Don't assume that doctors have only one office location. Initially, I hadn't asked receptionists if my doctors also worked in another town, and the receptionists did not bring it up. It's always good to ask what locations are available. Ask what days and times each doctor is at the various locations. If a doctor is only at a certain area once a month, but you'll need to see the doctor in that location weekly, that obviously will not work out. If the doctor you initially requested doesn't have a location close to you, perhaps another reputable doctor does.

If you think that you will want to see the same doctor at multiple locations, ask the receptionist about that. Some offices told me they prefer that I choose one location and stick with it, so they do not have to frequently transfer my records from one location to another. If you want to visit another location occasionally, I don't think transferring records would be problematic. You need to discuss such situations with each office.

Ask the office if they have a cancellation list.

If you were only able to get an appointment that is several months away from when you wanted it, ask the office if they will notify you if an opening arises. Some offices have a cancellation list and can add your name to it. If another patient cancels an appointment, the office will call and offer you that time slot.

If the office allows it, book far in advance to get an appointment slot that you want.

Some people prefer to schedule their appointments for the summer because it's easier for them to get out in the warmer weather. It can get tricky maintaining a summer schedule; for example, if you see a doctor in July for an annual visit, the doctor may ask you to return in one year. The receptionist, however, might tell you that no appointments are available until much later in the year. Or there might be a few openings, but not on the days or times you are available. You could thus end up on a fall or winter schedule. That's happened to me quite frequently. To avoid that problem, call the office months before your annual visit to set up your appointment for the following year. Booking earlier will increase your chances of getting an appointment when you want it.

If the doctor told you that it is very important that he or she see you within a specific timeframe, tell the receptionist, who will probably find a way to get you in sooner.

Avoid scheduling an appointment on days your doctor performs surgery.

If you want to increase the chances of your doctor being on time, it's best to avoid scheduling an appointment for a day he or she performs surgery. I once booked an appointment for one o'clock, not knowing that it was a day my doctor had to perform surgeries in the morning. The doctor was two hours late to my appointment due to unexpected circumstances during a surgery. At another facility, my doctor was delayed five hours for the same reason. I'm not complaining that the doctors were late; sometimes they can't avoid it. Emergencies can arise at any time, but they are probably more likely to occur on surgical days.

Some doctors do not have specific days of the week that they perform surgery; their schedules might vary. My experience is that offices usually know the surgical schedule at least two months in advance.

Your wait for your doctor might be less when you have the first appointment of the day or right after an office's lunch break.

When I've had the first appointment of the day or the first appointment after lunch, my wait time has been less for a doctor to come into the examining room. This has not always been the case, but most of the time it was. On one occasion, even though I had the first appointment of the day, I still had to wait quite a while because the doctor had scheduled a meeting. By mid-morning, doctors can lose bits of time because of phone calls, interruptions, unexpected delays, and patients who arrive late. Those bits of time add up throughout the day, making it difficult for a doctor to keep on schedule.

Be patient on the phone with receptionists. Be clear about the purpose of your appointment.

Be patient if you are put on hold when a receptionist answers the phone. If the wait is long, the good thing may be that the receptionist is not rushing the other person that they are talking to. That signals that you may not be rushed through your call either. Waiting is worthwhile when the receptionist is giving each caller good service.

Tell the receptionist the reason you are setting up an appointment. The receptionist will then have an idea of how much time you'll need with the doctor. If you want to talk to the doctor about a problem with your leg, request that a disability form be completed, and have x-rays examined, you should tell the receptionist. As you'll see later in this book, however, the reality is that you may not have enough time at your visit to cover everything you intended to. The receptionist can at least try to give you an extended appointment, if necessary.

Ask the office if they allow walk-in scheduling.

Some offices don't want you to walk into their office to schedule an appointment. I resorted to that several times when I could not get through on the phone. When I got to the office, the receptionist kept me waiting while she took phone calls from others who were also scheduling appointments. I got the feeling that she felt my presence was rather intrusive. If the office has only one or two workers, it can become problematic for them to handle walk-in schedulers. This is especially true if the person treating you is the only person there to answer the phone. Some places will check their answering machine between appointments. Ask your practitioners how they handle scheduling of appointments, and respect their rules.

Ask the receptionist to clarify the exact time of your follow-up appointment.

Receptionists should be trained to repeat the appointment date and time back to patients. That will avoid errors due to miscommunication. It's also reassuring to patients.

When booking follow-up appointments, some receptionists might tell you that your appointment is fifteen minutes earlier than it really is. I've asked some receptionists why they do this. One said she always tells everyone fifteen minutes earlier to be sure they arrive on time. She said many patients show up late, which throws off the doctor's schedule. Some receptionists neglect to tell their coworkers that they tell patients to arrive early. On a few occasions, at one particular office I showed up at my appointment fifteen minutes prior to my scheduled time. The receptionist that greeted me, however, said my appointment was actually fifteen minutes later than I was originally told. That resulted in my being thirty minutes early. Apparently, the receptionist that had booked me never told her coworkers that she didn't tell me the true time of my appointment.

Accept that your doctor may not walk into the room at your scheduled time.

I've experienced many mix-ups with appointments over the years. I've gotten to know what to expect from each office that I go to. If I book a nine o'clock appointment at some places, I know that the doctor will not actually see me until approximately nine thirty. With other offices, a nine o'clock appointment might mean that the doctor probably won't see me until ten o'clock.

You still need to show up on time. If you accept that your appointment may start late, you won't get so stressed out about it. If you have to see another doctor that same day, don't schedule both appointments too close to each other, in terms of time. If the first one runs late, you might be late for your other appointment.

Check with your insurance company to see if your visit is covered.

Sometimes, when making an appointment for an annual exam, the receptionist might tell you that your insurance will not pay unless it's been exactly a year since your last visit. You need to call your insurance company to find out if that matters. On several occasions, a receptionist told me that my insurance carrier would not cover my visit until a certain period of time had elapsed. The insurance company, however, told me that it would. Will you even have the same insurance the following year? If not, then having to wait exactly one year probably won't matter.

For follow-up appointments, ask the receptionist to write the date and time of your appointment on a card for you.

When you are at an office making a follow-up appointment, ask the receptionist to write the date and time of your next appointment on an appointment card. Bring it with you to your next appointment. While sitting in waiting rooms, I've overheard receptionists telling patients they did not have an appointment. The patients were insisting they had made the appointment, but they had not brought the appointment card to prove it.

I imagine that appointment cards will eventually become obsolete because so many procedures are being computerized. Some offices allow patients to schedule visits online. If you are offered the opportunity to schedule online, print out any e-mail confirmation that you receive, and bring it with you to your appointment.

Ask labs if they will allow you to schedule an appointment for your test.

Some labs allow you to make an appointment. I went to a lab early in the morning for a blood test and was the first person to walk in the door. Clients who arrived after I had, however, were taken first. I discovered they had made appointments. If such a convenience is important to you, ask your lab if it offers appointments. I now make appointments, and the process has worked out very well for me.

Don't rely on answering machines or a promise that someone will call you back.

When you call to make appointments, receptionists might tell you that they must call you back because they are busy. Sometimes they forget to call you back, or they don't have time to call you back that day. I usually respond by telling receptionists that they can call me, but that I may try to reach them later too. That leaves it open for me to call them, if too many hours go by without a call. If my call is not returned for several hours, how do I know if the receptionist forgot to call me back or was just not ready to call me yet?

It would be helpful if receptionists would tell patients that they might not be called back until much later in the day, or even the next day, if they know that's a possibility. That way, patients do not have to be concerned that the receptionist forgot to call them back. It's especially frustrating if, while waiting for their call, another patient reaches the office first and gets the time slot you wanted.

Sometimes you will have to leave a message on an answering machine. Some practitioners (not physicians) told me they do not always listen to their messages each day. Often, their answering systems did not say when they would return to the office. With most offices, I avoid leaving a message on an answering system. I prefer to keep calling until I get someone.

Some offices are great about returning calls in a timely manner. You will get to know the patterns of each office. If you have a rather urgent issue that is not an emergency, most answering systems will allow you to mark your message as urgent so that your call will quickly get attended to. Otherwise, it might immediately connect you to someone.

When Was the Last Time You Saw Your Doctors?

Don't let too much time elapse between visits to your doctors.

It's good to touch base periodically with your family doctor and specialists. Then, if you have a medical emergency, the doctors will have your recent history. One receptionist told me that, because I hadn't been to that particular office in several years, I would be considered a new patient. It resulted in my having to wait several months for an appointment. Ask offices how frequently you need to come in to remain an active patient in their files.

Be aware of administrative service fees.

Some doctors charge patients an annual fee to help cover the costs for time spent on administrative tasks.[5] Doctors and their staff spend excessive time on services for which they are not reimbursed, such as completing forms, transmitting records, and calling in referrals. Ask the receptionist if your doctor has administrative fees and for what services.

Length of Appointments

If you want an extended appointment, ask the receptionist to recommend a time slot most likely to ensure that you will get that much time during your visit.

I've sometimes booked extended appointments to allow more time with my doctor. Only occasionally did a specialist spend the allotted time with me. Once, a nurse told me I'd have to wait quite a while in the examining room before the doctor had time to see me for such a long appointment. When the doctor finally came into the room, he told me he only had ten minutes. Another time, my doctor was running fifteen minutes behind schedule. I knew that would probably mean that she was not going to give me the full thirty minutes that I had booked for my appointment; my assumption was correct. It's very frustrating when you had planned to have time to talk about various issues and then get rushed through the visit. On the other hand, I can understand the dilemma that doctors face when they are tight on time.

Long appointments can backfire for other reasons, too. Some practitioners take longer to do tasks because they know they have so much time to fill. Then you may still end up not getting everything covered that you intended to.

One of my biggest pet peeves is not having enough time at each visit to go over what I want. I've had numerous short appointments in which little was accomplished. Even my initial appointments were not long enough to fully go over my history.

Time would be better spent by a long initial appointment where a proper plan is set in place. Short initial visits can result in incorrect diagnoses and improper treatment plans. Short visits can also result in patients having to schedule follow-up appointments to cover everything they had hoped to address during the previous appointment.

My experience is that some practitioners are not realistic about the amount of time that patients need for follow-up appointments. Some practitioners told me they could do a certain task in ten minutes, but it usually took them double that time. When practitioners rush, they are prone to making errors, and their patients' visits will not be thorough.

I believe that most practitioners do not want to rush patients along. Numerous factors must be taken into account. An emergency may come up that throws off a doctor's schedule. Patients who arrive late throw off the schedule for other patients. In between visits, doctors might have phone calls to make or take. Physicians also have a lot of paperwork to complete for insurance companies and patients. Some doctors are under the time constraints set by insurance companies, which may allow doctors only so much time with each patient.

I think insurance companies would save money, in the long run, by allowing more time for office visits. Then, effective treatment plans can be established. Otherwise, unnecessary tests and procedures might be given.

Confirming Appointments

Ask what the procedure is to confirm appointments.

Offices differ in how they handle the confirmation of appointments. Some want the patient to call to confirm. Other offices are surprised if a patient initiates the confirmation, and some offices may not think it's necessary to confirm appointments. Some places want you to confirm the day before your appointment. Others want you to confirm two days before. One office typically left me messages to confirm my appointment in which it also stated that I must call back to confirm I got the message. Some offices assume that patients know how the office handles confirmation procedures. Offices should discuss that with patients when they arrive for their initial appointment. If receptionists don't tell you what their procedures are, ask.

If your doctor has offices in several locations, confirm the specific location of your appointment. If you scheduled an appointment far in advance, I suggest confirming it periodically. If in January, I book an appointment for September, I confirm it in April to be sure it's still in the books and that the doctor has not changed his or her schedule. I call again as the date gets closer.

When you call to confirm an appointment, a receptionist might tell you that your name is not on the schedule. If you don't speak up, you may lose an appointment that you had really made. You need to be assertive and tell the receptionist you are certain that you booked it. It's helpful if you can say when you booked the appointment and the name of the worker who scheduled it. Sometimes, after receptionists look a little deeper in their computer systems, they find it.

These days, many confirmations are handled via an automatic phone message sent to your home. This is efficient and usually works out pretty well. Once, however, after I pressed the button to confirm an appointment, the system didn't acknowledge it. It repeatedly asked me to confirm my appointment. I called the office the next day to confirm the appointment and to report that the answering system was not working correctly. If you are not certain that an automated system got your message, call the office during normal business hours and ask.

I experienced another issue regarding the confirmation of appointments. A doctor's office gave me an appointment card that said my appointment was scheduled for 9:30. I was told that I'd have a test at 9:30 and then be hooked up to equipment that I was to wear home. A week prior to my appointment, I confirmed it for 9:30. Two days before my appointment, an automated message stated that my appointment was scheduled for 10:15. It also said that I should arrive fifteen minutes early. I called the office to see why the automated system said 10:15 instead of 9:30. The person who answered the phone said the automated system was confirming the time that I was scheduled to be hooked up to the equipment. I wondered why I had not previously been told that my being hooked up to a machine was given a separate appointment time of 10:15. I also wondered how I could arrive fifteen minutes early, if I was still undergoing the other test right before it. This example shows how you must call the office if there is any doubt about an appointment time. If I hadn't questioned my situation, I might have shown up 10:15 for the appointment and missed a portion of it. It also shows how an office should be thorough in explaining appointment and confirmation procedures.

You'd be surprised at the changes in schedules that can arise before your appointment. If practitioners cancel you at the last minute, you'll sometimes have to wait a long time for another appointment. Some receptionists confirmed my appointments, but when I arrived at the office they told me that I never scheduled one. Some receptionists might switch your appointment to another date but forget to tell you.

Doctors with Multiple Locations

Be sure your file is at the same office location as your visit.

If you don't always go to the same office location, ask the receptionist if he or she needs to transfer your file to the office where you will be seen. Some of my doctors were disappointed when they found out that my file was not there. Call a few days before your appointment to be sure that your file is in the appropriate office. The office staff may find you intrusive for checking, but you have to look out for yourself. Often receptionists assured me that my file would be transferred to the appropriate office on time, but when I got to my appointment it wasn't there.

Traveling Long Distance to a Doctor

Consider an out-of-state doctor, but don't think that traveling far will necessarily give you what you need.

You might think you can get better care outside of your local area. Don't assume that just because you travel far, the visit will be any more beneficial than with a local doctor. It can be, but not necessarily. I've had just as many good and bad visits by traveling great distances as I have had locally. I even had local doctors question why I traveled so far to see a doctor. They seemed suspicious about it, for some reason.

Rescheduling Appointments

Use caution when rescheduling appointments.

Sometimes, when I had rescheduled appointments, receptionists forgot to put the change in their computer system; so when I called months later to confirm my appointment, they said I never booked it. I now confirm my appointments way ahead of time and also a few days prior to the appointment. I want to be sure that nothing got messed up.

Occasionally your doctor's office may have to reschedule your appointment. The office staff may not realize how changing appointments can be a problem for patients who have to reschedule rides or arrange time off from work. If you frequently cancel and reschedule rides, the facility that provides your transportation may not think so highly of you. Situations do come up that shift a doctor's schedule around, however, which can't be avoided. If you tell a receptionist that you cannot switch your appointment, sometimes he or she will say that is okay. The receptionist might just be trying to shift your appointment because another patient wanted the time you had. If you let the office change your appointment, the other person will be happy, but you won't be. When a receptionist calls me to reschedule, I usually ask why the change is necessary. The answer keys me in as to how much leeway I have in trying to keep my original appointment. I try to look at the whole picture and be fair.

If you have a chronic illness, you may need to see various specialists frequently. Setting up multiple appointments can become exhausting, especially if rescheduling occurs. You can ask the receptionist and your practitioner to avoid rescheduling you, unless absolutely necessary. Other patients may not mind having their appointments switched and may be more flexible than you.

Patients should also be considerate of an office's situation. Don't make a habit of frequently rescheduling. Plan your schedule ahead of time the best that you can.

Cancellations

Be aware that your appointment might suddenly be canceled, even after you recently confirmed it.

My sister traveled all the way from Pennsylvania to bring our mother, who was in a nursing home, to an appointment. My mother's 10:00 appointment was confirmed by the nursing home at approximately 9:15, just before my mother left the nursing home. When my mother and sister arrived at the doctor's office, the receptionist told them that the doctor got called to an emergency while they were traveling. You can imagine all that my mother and the nursing staff had gone through to get my mother ready for the appointment.

I once had an appointment at a local office for noontime. I confirmed it right before I left the house. My traveling time was about thirty minutes. When I arrived at the office, the receptionist said that my appointment was suddenly canceled because the manager decided to have a meeting with her staff.

I had a similar situation with another appointment, for which my husband took a vacation day off from work to take me there. I confirmed the appointment the day before. The morning of the appointment, a secretary called me and said my practitioner was conducting a meeting and that I'd have to see someone else at the facility. I was disappointed because I had made my original appointment with someone that another practitioner had recommended.

Ask the office to explain its cancellation policy.

The first time you visit an office, find out its cancellation policy. If it requires a twenty-four hour notice, and you don't give one, it has the right to charge you. If a medical or family emergency arises that causes you to cancel, tell the office. Some offices are understanding in those situations and may bend the rules, especially if it's your first time canceling. Don't take advantage of the cancellation policy by pretending you had an emergency when you didn't.

Remote Consultations

Consider asking doctors if they offer phone consultations.

I was fortunate to have a holistic doctor who allowed phone consultations. I've been very happy with the phone consultations that I received. Usually, it's important that the initial visit be done in the office. The ability to be allowed a phone consultation depends upon your affliction. Phone consultations are especially helpful if the office is far away or if you can't drive. I've gotten a great deal accomplished with phone consultations. They covered many details and in a shorter timeframe than my office visits; furthermore, there were no distractions. My phone consultations have never been paid for by insurance.

I think phone consultations, web-based consultations, and various types of remote consultations will become common.

Directions

Don't always rely on the office staff for directions.

Many people have a GPS system in their car or use of the Internet, so obtaining good directions to their doctor's office is not much of an issue. Those who don't have a GPS or computer may have to rely on the office staff for directions. I was surprised to find that many offices do not have written directions to their facility for clients. When you ask receptionists for directions, you'll find that some are better at giving directions than others. It would be helpful if receptionists could at least give clients accurate directions from major highways. One office mailed me directions, which I really appreciated. Some places have directions on their phone answering system or website.

Find out where the parking facilities are, prior to your visit.

When scheduling your initial appointment, ask the office where their parking facilities are located and whether parking is free. Parking is often very close to the facility. Sometimes, though, you may be surprised how far the parking lot is from an office. If you park in a hospital parking garage, you might need to cross over a walkway, which can be quite a distance from the office. When scheduling your appointment, ask the office if handicapped parking, wheelchair ramps, wheelchairs, or scooters are available if you need them. If the parking is quite a distance from the actual office, ask for specific directions from the parking area to the facility.

Transport Services

Know the ins and outs of using transportation services.

Some patients are not able to drive, whether for temporary or permanent reasons. They may need to arrange for transportation with Dial-A-Rides, paratransit services, taxis, friends, family members, or even limos. I have had to use many of these services at times. I've noticed that people mistakenly use the term Dial-A-Ride and paratransit interchangeably. In the geographic area where I live, the Dial-A-Ride service is a bit limited as far as what days of the week and what times it takes people to medical appointments. Not all towns have a Dial-A-Ride, and the age requirements might vary from town to town. The paratransit service in my area is offered to those who meet certain physical impairments according to the American with Disabilities Act. It operates daily. Its weekend hours, however, differ from weekdays. The availability of paratransit services can depend upon where you live. The paratransit service where I live usually charges a fee; however, because of the town in which I am a resident, I am able to use the services for free. Whether or not you are charged a fee might depend upon where you live. I use the term Dial-A-Ride and paratransit interchangeably in the following sections, but just for the ease of reading. My comments that follow would apply to either the Dial-A-Ride or paratransit services, anyway.

Although I appreciate the transit services, using them is not as easy as many think. It's challenging to figure out when to tell your ride to pick you up from an appointment. It's difficult to judge how long you will be at an appointment, since you don't know how long you will have to wait for the doctor. Some Dial-A-Ride services have a policy of arriving within fifteen minutes before, or after, the time they are scheduled to get you. If you have a 1:00 appointment, you'd have to take into account that the appointment may not really start until 1:30. You then have to guess how long the appointment will be and what time to tell your driver to pick you up. You also have to take into account that if you tell Dial-A-Ride to pick you up at 3:00, they will get you any time between 2:45 and 3:15. It's frustrating, because you can end up sitting at facilities for an hour or more, just waiting for your ride. Bring a book or something to do while you are waiting. Plan your appointment times and rides in a way that avoids your getting stuck at an office after closing time.

At some facilities, it's hard to see if your ride is approaching. Some offices might not have a window nearby. If you have to use a bathroom at a facility while waiting for your ride, it can get tricky. Some Dial-A-Rides allow their drivers to wait only five minutes for the person being picked up. If your doctor's office has a bathroom down the hall, if you need a key for the bathroom, or if the bathroom is on another level, you can miss your ride by the time you get out of the bathroom. Some facilities do not have any place to sit while you wait by a door for your ride.

If you are waiting at a large medical complex with multiple entrances and exits, the driver might not know where to find you. When scheduling an appointment for the ride, give the operator a tip as to where the driver will be able to locate you. The scheduler may be able to input that tip into the computer system to make it easier for the driver to spot you. Some services might offer to call you on your cell phone soon before they will arrive.

After my medical and dental appointments, some receptionists have offered to call the Dial-A-Ride service to say I'm ready to be picked up. Some receptionists don't realize, however, that most ride services cannot be expected to respond so quickly. I appreciate that the offices try to help me out, but it only complicates matters sometimes. There might be occasions when a Dial-A-Ride driver suggests that you call if you finish early, in case he or she is available. I've found their ability to get me quickly was rare and not to be expected.

I've been in some Dial-a-Ride vehicles in which the ride was very bumpy and uncomfortable. I've been in many vehicles in which the seat belts do not tighten enough for thin people. If you find that the seat belts do not fit you correctly, inform the service that provided the ride. Others and I have had a few occasions in which our driver never showed up. If your ride hasn't shown up within the timeframe it should have, call the ride service. It could be that the vehicle broke down or that the driver is lost.

When boarding a transport service vehicle, if you tell the driver that you know the best route to your destination, the driver will not know how much to trust you for giving good directions. Poor directions can cause the driver great delays. Some drivers appreciate help with directions and others don't. You will get to know the drivers over time. They also will get to know how much they can trust you to give accurate directions. It's obviously not your job to give the driver directions, but it can be helpful to tell them of routes that they may not have known about. Some drivers are more pleasant than others, and some are better drivers than others, no matter what service you use. Some special transit services require the driver to walk you to the door of the medical facility, or at least wait until you get inside the facility. If the drivers are not doing their job, report it to the facility that provided you with the ride. Before you use a service, ask what procedures the drivers should be following when clients enter and exit their vehicles.

I wish all transit services would train their drivers about invisible illnesses. Drivers may not realize the nature of your affliction, if they can't see it, and be less likely to walk you to the door.

If you need to use special transit services because you have a walking impairment, your doctor will usually have to complete a form to verify why you need the service. You must meet certain qualifications for those services. Some services may also want to interview you in person, prior to you using their services.

In addition to transit services, I've also taken taxis. A taxi service that I used had very cramped seating in the back of the cab. I could barely stand the ride home because the back seat area was very confining. I'm very small, and I can imagine that an average-sized person would feel even more uncomfortable than I did. I called the manager of the cab company to tell him that I was very uncomfortable in the back. He suggested that I tell drivers that I want to sit in the front and to mention that I had talked to the manager. The driver can make the final call as to whether he or she trusts someone to sit in the front. I tried the manager's suggestion on my next ride, and it worked fine.

Rarely has a taxi shown up on time for me. There are not a lot of taxi services in my local area. Some require that you book the ride at least four hours before you want the taxi to arrive. One place wanted me to schedule the ride the day before I needed it. Some cab drivers who've picked me up have arrived more than an hour late. Waiting can get very difficult if you have to stand outside for the driver to spot you. Some drivers went right past me, despite my waving to signal them. For those reasons, I avoid using taxis. Occasionally a cab driver will call you on your cell just before he or she arrives, if you tell them to. Some people live in areas where they can easily grab a cab. If so, they are fortunate if it works out well for them. If the service you use is not adequate, call and suggest how to improve the service. If enough people complain, perhaps companies will make positive changes in their services.

Have you ever used a limo to go places? I have, and it was quite humorous. I felt like a queen. I use limos when a doctor's office is too far away for me to take the Dial-A-Ride. The limo drivers I had were very pleasant and made the rides enjoyable.

If friends or acquaintances are driving you, ask them if they want gas money. Try to use a driver whose company you like, because you don't want the ride to be a negative experience. I always tell my drivers that my appointment is a bit earlier than it actually is, because some drivers cut time a bit too close for my comfort. I usually need time to go over paperwork when I arrive at an office, and I may want to use the bathroom. I like to be on time for my appointments, so I allow time for unexpected delays on the road. Some drivers will sit with you through an appointment. Others may want to drop you off and pick you up later. I usually tell friends to pick me up thirty minutes later than I think my appointment will end; otherwise, I arrange to call when I'm ready.

❦❦❦❦

Obstacles upon Arrival
at the Facility

Unmaintained Parking Lots

Be prepared for unmaintained lots.

I often notice that sidewalks outside of medical facilities are not shoveled, even when there was ample time to clear the snow. Practitioners rarely own the lots. It's the lot owner's responsibility to maintain the lot. Clients might think a staff member could at least go out and shovel a small path. But this could raise liability issues. A receptionist, for example, is hired for specific duties that do not usually include shoveling snow. One would think a lot owner would take great care to keep the lot clear to avoid liability issues.

If you think a parking lot is not adequately maintained, report it to the lot owner. You can usually find out who owns a lot by calling your town hall. Perhaps your practitioner will know who the lot owner is. Some owners live out of the local area and may not even be aware of the situation.

During the winter, I schedule most of my appointments for early afternoon when the temperatures are usually warmer. I avoid late afternoon appointments because sidewalks often ice up when the sun begins to set. Sometimes, I carry a small bag of sand and toss the sand as I walk.

Stuck Outside

When scheduling your appointments, ask about the availability of restrooms.

Some places might tell you that they have a bathroom. When you arrive at their facility, however, the doors to the building might be locked if it's early in the morning. If your practitioner is prone to being late and you have the first appointment of the day, you may be left outside waiting. This is a problem for patients who have bladder issues or other medical conditions. Inquire about the availability of an office's restroom facilities when you are scheduling your initial appointment.

Upon arrival to an appointment for a massage one winter, I had to wait outside. I had told the massage therapist about my bladder problem, and she assured me there was a bathroom at the facility. When I arrived, I noticed a sign hanging on her outside door that said "Session in Progress." The door was locked, and it was very cold outside. I waited a while in my car with the heater on.

Eventually I had to find a bathroom, so I drove to a supermarket to use the one there. When I returned, the door was still locked, and the sign was still up. I waited approximately fifteen minutes more, then left. To my surprise, the massage therapist later called me at home and was mad at me for leaving. It was just poor customer service on her part not to forewarn me of the situation, especially knowing about my bladder condition. It never dawned on me that a practitioner's "waiting room" could be outside!

On another occasion, a massage therapist told me there was a bathroom down the hall from his office that I could use when he was in. He told me that he might arrive late, but not to worry since there was another doctor in the building whose bathroom I could use if I had to. The massage therapist failed to tell me that the doctor was not at the facility every day of the week. If I arrived early on days that doctor was not in or my massage therapist was late, I would be stuck waiting with no available bathroom. I might also have been stuck outside if the door to the main building was locked.

I have run into such problems at other practitioners' offices, as well.

Accessible Parking

Educate the public about obstacles to handicapped parking.

If you qualify for a handicapped parking permit, be sure to apply for one. Most states allow you to apply for either a temporary or permanent permit, depending on your need. Some may charge a small fee. It took me months to get the courage to apply for the permit because I didn't want to admit that I had a problem walking. I should have applied sooner. I had suffered needlessly trying to walk distances that were very difficult for me. I obtained an application for a handicapped parking permit through the Department of Motor Vehicles. My doctor had to complete the application and specify why I needed the permit. State laws and processes may vary. You must meet certain impairment requirements to be approved for the permit. Some people can apply for a special handicapped license plate instead of a hanging placard. Keep that in mind if you notice a car in a handicapped space that does not have a hanging placard.

I was surprised that I was issued a lifetime permit. What if my condition later changed for the better? People should be assessed periodically to be sure they still require the permit. Otherwise, they might use a permit that they no longer need. Fortunately, my state now requires more frequent checking and periodic approvals.

Getting the permit is only half the battle. You then must be lucky enough to find an available handicapped parking space. The following are obstacles that I have noticed regarding handicapped parking spaces:

- Some drivers park over the cross-hatch, which is for wheelchair access. Either the driver did not take care to properly park in the space, or two cars with handicapped permits parked in one handicapped space. (The cross-hatch consists of the diagonal lines to the sides of the space).

- Drivers without handicapped permits illegally park in the spaces. I have become a bit daring in approaching those drivers and asking them to move their cars. This is risky, because you never know how the person will react. Use caution if you confront a driver. Always be polite.

- Some handicapped spaces merely have a handicapped sign painted on the pavement, without an accompanying above-ground sign. When it snows and the sign on the pavement is covered, drivers can't distinguish the handicapped spaces.

- Handicapped spaces are often the least plowed. Those spaces are usually in corners and prone to piles of snow from the plows. Some lot owners have told me that the signs impede their plowing efforts. This is a valid concern, yet alternate methods of clearing the snow could be used. The problem results in the handicapped spaces being the least accessible spaces in the parking lot.

- Some people use the handicapped parking area as a place to leave their shopping carts. I have seen carts left there by those with and without handicapped parking permits. Some of this may be due to laziness, but we must also consider that many people with handicapped permits might be too fatigued to return their carts. It would be helpful if there was a defined area near the handicapped spaces for carts.

- Some people use a deceased relative's handicapped parking permit or borrow someone else's permit. A family member or other responsible party should return a permit once the original holder has passed away. You should not borrow permits from another person to use as your own.

- Some people continue to use their handicapped parking permit beyond its expiration date, even though they no longer have a walking impairment. Permits should be returned once you no longer have the walking impairment.

- Some handicapped spaces are on treacherous slopes. There is a legal limit to slopes. If you think a slope is too steep, inform the lot owner.

- Those with invisible impairments are often yelled at by others who think they are misusing the space. I try to react calmly to such people. On the one hand, I know they are watching out for abusers of the space. On the other hand, it's rude of them to yell. Many with heart disease, lung disease, fibromyalgia, multiple sclerosis, and numerous other conditions may not look impaired. A person might have severe fatigue or pain when they are walking that is not visible to others. Some people might start out walking normally but suddenly get fatigued.

- Some people who are young, or look young, are yelled at by others who think they are too young to be disabled. Age does not prevent a person from having impairments.

- Delivery truck drivers often park in the spaces to unload items. I talked to a mailman who did not have a handicapped permit, but who I saw repeatedly use the spaces. After I confronted him, he stopped parking in the handicapped spaces. He may have also been concerned that I would report him if he didn't comply.

- A local police department told me they don't have much time to check parking lots for offenders of handicapped parking spaces.

- Some lot owners put up special parking spaces for seniors and expectant mothers. In some of those lots, I noticed they took away one or two handicapped parking spaces. Even if done in a legal manner, I question the fairness of this. If pregnancy is severely impairing a woman's ability to walk, perhaps she should apply for a temporary handicapped permit.

- Some stores have their handicapped spaces very close to their entrances. Their exits, however, may be at the opposite end of the building. That results in the handicapped spaces being very far away upon exiting these stores.

There are many things you can do to help alleviate the obstacles. Some towns have programs for volunteers to work with local police in ticketing those who park illegally. Volunteer groups could be established to educate the public about these obstacles. I believe that many people don't realize the impact they have when they misuse handicapped parking spaces.

If you think a lot is not conforming to the current handicapped parking laws, contact the lot owner, whose identity might be found at town hall. You can spread awareness of the issues through the media. You can be a good example, too, by respecting the spaces and not abusing them. You can write editorials in newspapers, suggest articles for magazines, or initiate a radio show in which you speak about the problems. You can ask disability advocacy groups to create a brochure about obstacles to the handicapped parking spaces. Get permission to distribute the brochures at hospitals, colleges, senior centers, and health fairs.

It is critical that our educational system be a part of this awareness. Children could be taught respect for the spaces at a young age using, for instance, puppets. Driver education classes should incorporate the issue of handicapped parking into their curriculum. Departments of Motor Vehicles could offer classes in which they discuss the issues. They usually note something briefly in their brochures, but the information in my state's brochure is not very extensive. There is so much we can do as individuals, and as a group.

The Handicapped Parking Symbol

Brainstorm how the international handicapped parking symbol can be changed to reflect invisible disabilities, too.

There is a great need for a new symbol to represent handicapped parking. Because there is just a wheelchair symbol on a handicapped parking placard or license plate, others may think that someone walking without an assistive device should not be in the space. It's unfortunate to those suffering with invisible impairments. There should be a competition to redesign the international handicapped parking symbol to reflect invisible walking impairments too.

If you have any ideas for a new symbol, I suggest contacting the U.S. Department of Justice. You can ask staff there if they know who you can present your idea to.

(Handicapped parking is also known as accessible parking.)

Heavy Doors

If the doors at a particular facility are very heavy and hard to open, inform the staff.

Haven't we all come across heavy doors at a medical facility? It is an unfair challenge to battle a heavy door, especially while using crutches, a cane, a wheelchair, or other assistive device. It's also cumbersome for the person bringing someone in with a wheelchair. It's hard even for those without assistive devices who have bad backs, weak upper body strength, and other medical conditions. I've seen unfit patients politely trying to hold doors open for each other. It would be great if every office had a buzzer outside that patients could use to alert a staff worker when they need help opening the door. Functional automatic doors would be very helpful to patients, but they are costly to install in older buildings. Patients need to voice their opinions about heavy doors. If enough of us speak up, perhaps changes will be made.

Parking Garages

You might find that it's easier to get to the doctor's office by walking outside a parking garage rather than trying to locate it from the inside.

Sometimes, it's quicker to walk outside the parking garage to get to a doctor's office, as opposed to navigating it from inside the parking garage. I first realized this at a hospital. I had to walk over a bridge, down a few flights of steps, and then find my way through a maze of hallways. I finally discovered that if I had just walked outside the parking garage, I would have easily gotten to the office. Of course, in bad weather, an inside route is often best. You also have to watch for parked cars backing up, along with other traffic, inside the garage.

Inside the Office

Coat Racks

It's often easier to hang onto your coat than to use coat racks.

This may seem trivial, but some offices don't have enough places for patients to hang their coats. When the coat racks are full, some people place their coat on top of another person's coat. Patients with weak upper body strength can find it difficult to push through the layers of coats to find their own. I don't mind bringing my coat into an examining room with me during an appointment. In fact, I actually prefer that, since my coat was stolen or mistakenly taken from a coat rack once. If the treatment room is small, an office might prefer that coats be left in the waiting room.

Many offices have plants and other decorative furnishings by their coat racks, which can also make it difficult for patients to access the rack. The plants and furnishings look nice, but they may not be practical. Coat racks, in some offices, are not at a reasonable height for someone in a wheelchair to reach.

Clocks

Don't assume that the clocks in the office show the correct time.

Some practitioners purposely set their clocks ten minutes ahead to keep themselves on schedule. It's confusing for patients to see clocks set to different times. Sometimes clocks gain or lose time on their own and need to be reset. I've found many places are careless about checking and coordinating their clocks for the correct time.

Late Arrivals

Be respectful of time.

Do your best to arrive at your appointment on time. This is especially important if you are the first patient of the day or the first patient after the office's lunchtime. If you are late, it will throw off the doctor's schedule. Being on time is respectful to both doctors and other patients. It also sends a message that you care.

I think most patients don't get upset if their doctor is running late due to an emergency, or because another patient's visit is taking longer than anticipated. I am especially tolerant of this in orthopedic offices. Injuries come up unexpectedly, and it's probably difficult for a doctor to know how long it will take to treat each patient.

Time gets off track immediately when a practitioner arrives late to the office and starts the first appointment late. These little bits of time add up throughout the day. Before you know it, the practitioner is forty-five minutes or more behind. This is really not necessary if all would do their part to be respectful of time. I usually request the first appointment of the day with practitioners who have a habit of being late. That way, I'll probably only wait ten to fifteen minutes for them to arrive, as opposed to a much longer time as their delays accumulate throughout the day. I know some practitioners who run late and try to make it up by cutting each appointment by five to ten minutes. That's not fair to patients who were on time.

The Disadvantage of Arriving Early

Arriving too early for your appointment is sometimes not in your best interest.

If you arrive extremely early for an appointment, the staff may try to squeeze you in. Whenever I hear the term "squeeze," I cringe. That usually means my visit will be cut short. You can politely say that you'd prefer to wait. It can get a bit awkward, though, if they want you to be seen earlier than scheduled. At times, I was looking forward to being early because I had phone calls to make prior to my visit. I wanted to be relaxed and not rushed. I often find it best to wait in the hallway, if possible, to avoid such situations.

If you come in too early, it can give the impression that you have little else to do. This is especially true if you are on disability. It's very hard to judge the time you will arrive when you are using a Dial-A-Ride service or other transportation service. If you can drive yourself, consider that it's best to not arrive extremely early.

Windows and Paperwork

Your first welcome to the office may be a closed glass window.

One of my pet peeves is being greeted by a closed glass window at the check-in desk. Sometimes the receptionist is on the phone and doesn't even look up to acknowledge you. If the window is tinted, you can't even see if anyone is at the desk. I find the constant opening and closing of such windows distracting. It certainly is not welcoming to patients.

I have never asked an office the reason for a closed window. Perhaps it's so the receptionist has fewer distractions. It could be to keep the noise level down for patients and employees. It could also be for safety or privacy reasons.

Come prepared to complete your paperwork accurately, completely, neatly, and efficiently.

During your first visit to an office, you will be required to fill out forms regarding your medical history and the reason for your visit. You will also have privacy forms to sign.

When I make initial appointments, I ask receptionists if they will send me the paperwork ahead of time. That way, I can take my time filling it out and be sure that my answers are legible and correct. Some offices will agree to mail the paperwork, but others will want you to complete it on site. One office let me complete its forms online.

I don't like filling out the forms in the office for several reasons. My hands usually get too fatigued to fill in so much information at one sitting. Some forms do not have enough room on them for those with a lengthy history to fill in necessary information. I'm usually told to arrive fifteen minutes early to fill out the forms. Fifteen minutes may not be enough time for someone with several chronic conditions. Those with a lengthy medical history or whose hands get fatigued when writing, may need at least thirty minutes.

I think an office's lack of concern for this paperwork should be of major concern to patients. It is important that the forms be legible and that they accurately reflect your history, medications, allergies, insurance, and other critical information. When new patients are scheduling appointments, offices should tell them to bring in their medical history and a complete list of allergies.

Some receptionists assumed I had the same insurance plan as the prior year, despite my giving them a recent medical card. The insurance carrier was the same, but the account number and plan had changed. Apparently, some receptionists just looked at the insurance carrier name and assumed the plan had not changed. If the receptionists had thoroughly examined my medical card, they would have noticed the account number changed. Even when I verbally pointed out the change, some receptionists still ignored it. That resulted in some of my claims being denied. Be sure receptionists clearly understand what insurance plan(s) you have.

When I fill out forms at a doctor's office, I don't always complete them in the order of the questions. That's because receptionists usually don't allow me enough time to fully complete forms before I am called into the examining room. I try to fill in the most important areas first. I start with my name, date of birth, and the main purpose of my visit. I then complete the allergy and medical history sections. I complete the insurance and privacy forms last, because I know an office will give me time for them later. After my visit, I will ask to have a form back if I haven't fully completed it. At that point, some receptionists have told me it's not necessary to complete the rest of the form, unless it's to fill in the privacy or insurance information. I know the paperwork is a critical piece of information in my file, though, if it ever needed to be accessed. Insist that receptionists allow you to fully complete the forms.

Over time, I have realized that some of my doctors were just skimming over the forms that I completed. When I handed one doctor my form that I had spent an hour completing, he stuck it in the file without looking at it. During the visit, he kept asking me the same questions I had already answered on the form. I politely asked him why he didn't just look at the form. He said he has patients fill forms out in case he needs to refer to them in the future, but rarely looks at them except for allergies to medications. It is not uncommon for a staff worker, a nurse, and my doctor to all ask me what my allergies are, even though I already put that information on their form.

Some hospitals in the United States expedite the check-in process with a digital device that scans patients' palms to access health records.[6] A palm scan is taken and a profile made for each patient.[7] During subsequent visits a patient checks-in by putting his or her hand on the device.[8]

I think the use of palm scans is excellent as long as the initial profile is set up correctly.

Don't assume that an office will accept your typed or printed attachment to their form.

The issue of whether you can add your own attachment to a form varies from office to office. Because of my lengthy medical history, I usually bring in a typed list of my allergies, medications, and surgeries. In the areas of the form where it asks me to list my allergies, medications, and surgeries, I will write, "see attached." My typed list enables me to present the office with an accurate and legible history. Some offices would not accept my attachment because they didn't want extra paperwork. I then had to go back and quickly write the information on their form. Other offices appreciated my efforts. What one office likes, another may not.

If your doctor or a staff member inputs your medical history into a computer, verify that he or she has done so accurately.

Some doctors input information directly into a computer as they ask you specific questions during your visit, instead of having you complete a form. I don't like that method for several reasons. The doctors that input my information were barely glancing at me, since they were so focused on getting the information into the computer. This approach also steals discussion and evaluation time from the visit. Also, I am concerned about how accurately the information will be input if the person entering it is not detail-oriented, or doesn't understand what I said.

When an office worker was inputting my medical history into the computer, she asked me what medications I took. Unfortunately, I had forgotten to bring the name of a recent medication that I was given. She said that was okay. I told her it was not okay, since it was an important piece of information for my file. I told her that I'd call the office later with the information. At that same visit, I caught an error in the computer system, which listed that I was taking a medication that I never took.

Years ago, when computers were just becoming popular in offices, I was told my doctor's computer software did not have enough room to list all of my allergies. The receptionist said that was okay. When I got home, I typed a list of my allergies. I then mailed it to their office and asked that it be kept in my file.

It's not a bad idea to ask the person inputting your information to read it back to you to verify that they entered it correctly. I even ask them to spell back my medications.

If you have a change of insurance or new allergies, inform your doctor's office.

Offices will periodically ask you to update your insurance and allergy information. It's best, however, to inform your doctors' offices as soon as you know of a change, rather than waiting until your next visit. That way, if an emergency comes up before your next visit, the information will be in your file. If you have a new medical condition that is important for your doctors to know of, set up an appointment with your doctors. Keep your doctors informed.

Tiny Print on Insurance ID Cards

If the print on your insurance card is too small to read, inform your insurance carrier.

I know my eyes are not what they were when I was young, but the print on some medical ID cards is too small to read clearly. I usually have to get a magnifying glass out to see it. I don't understand why it has to be that tiny. Perhaps if enough of us complain to our insurance carriers about this, they will start enlarging the print. I wouldn't be surprised if these cards eventually have a code on them that can be read by a computer.

A pet peeve of mine is insurance carriers who do not issue dental insurance identification cards. Some carriers told me to show the dental office my medical card. This was confusing to the receptionists because the medical card did not list the dental plan or phone number. More recently, I have had plans that enable me to print dental cards online. I never understood why some carriers don't issue dental cards. Perhaps it's a cost issue.

Multiple Insurance Carriers

Inform the office about all of your insurances. If you know the proper order of which plan pays first, tell the receptionist.

It is imperative that you inform receptionists about all of your insurance plans and whether you are the primary insured on the plan, or a dependent. You also need to tell them if you are retired, on disability, or actively working, as that will make a difference as to which insurance plan pays first. The number of employees at your or your spouse's employer is sometimes important, as well. Various factors will contribute to which insurance carrier pays first and how the benefits are coordinated.

If you have multiple carriers, be certain you know the correct order of which insurance plan pays first. You should find that out by calling all of your health insurance carriers. Be sure that all insurance carriers agree on the proper order of payment, and ask them to send you a letter to confirm the order in writing. They may not agree to send you something in writing, but it's worth asking. Communicate the order very clearly to receptionists. I've found that many offices submitted to the wrong carrier first, despite my telling them the correct order. Those claims had to be redone, which meant I had to wait longer to get money that was due to me.

Take the order of payment seriously, especially if Medicare is involved. Medicare follows its guidelines very strictly, and it will ask for any money back that it should not have paid out. For many years, my insurance carriers told me what they thought was the proper order of payment for my claims. Then one of my carriers questioned which insurance carrier should be the primary payer of my claims, and contacted Medicare about it. This ultimately led to Medicare demanding that all of my claims from several years ago be redone, and insisting on getting money back that it should not have paid.

Medicare held my husband's employer, through whom we had medical insurance, responsible. Apparently, when my husband first started working for this employer, they had a certain number of employees. At some point, this number of employees increased, but my husband didn't know that. The number of employees had an impact upon which insurance plan would pay first. The incident was a nightmare, and certainly another added stress, not only for my husband and me, but also for my doctors.

Years later, Medicare and our insurance carriers questioned the order of payment again, even after they had supposedly resolved it. Fortunately, I had requested letters from the carriers about the proper order when the issue arose the first time. I still had their letters, so I sent copies to the insurance carriers to prove that the issue was already settled. That resulted in the insurance companies finally putting the issue to rest. It's hard to find people with the skill and experience who know the order of which insurance carrier pays first. You begin to wonder who really knows the correct procedures.

Loud Staff and Private Issues

If receptionists or other staff members are talking too loud about your personal information, ask them to please keep their voices down.

I think that some receptionists don't realize how loud they talk when discussing personal information with patients. Likewise, some patients may not realize how loud they are when answering questions. Often, patients are asked about their Social Security number, insurance identification number, birth date, and physical ailments. In some offices, I can hear what a doctor is saying to a patient when they are in a private room. You have to be especially careful of this in treatment areas with no walls.

Perhaps staff members could take patients to a private area to check-in. That would alleviate any concerns about other people in the waiting room overhearing a patient's personal matters.

Fortunately, the issue of personal information being overheard will diminish as palm scans are incorporated into more facilities.

The Risks of Being Friendly with the Staff

Use caution if you form friendships with the staff.

Over time, it's natural to build up a certain rapport with the staff. At some point, you may be in a situation where an office worker didn't handle something about your care correctly. You know you need to stand up for yourself. You also know that if you confront the office worker about the issue, you will risk your relationship with that person and perhaps the entire office. Several patients have told me they don't bring issues up because they don't want to cause any friction. Sometimes, though, you need to risk the relationship to get what you deserve. Otherwise, you are giving the office staff an easy out. You have to let go of wanting people to like you all the time. Confrontations can be especially awkward if you have built up a good business relationship with one of the staff members.

Privacy

Realize that the Health Insurance Portability and Accountability Act (HIPAA) Privacy Rule is not as clear-cut as it seems.

The HIPAA Privacy Rule has national standards to protect the privacy of your health care information.[9] For more information about HIPAA regulations, go to www.hhs.gov.[10] HIPAA is an extremely complex federal law. If you feel your privacy rights were violated, consider talking with an attorney or contacting the U.S. Department of Health and Human Services.

I once tried to prevent a dentist from sharing my dental records with another dentist. This did not go over well and made the dentist suspicious of me. I called a dental office to tell them that I'd like to make an appointment as a new patient. I told the secretary that I did not want their dentist to notify my regular dentist about my appointment. The receptionist said that she would call me back after discussing that issue with dentists in that office. She called me later to tell me that one of the dentists said he would not see me unless I allowed him to share the information with my primary dentist. He thought that sharing the information was critical to my care. So, they gave me an appointment with another dentist in the practice who agreed to honor my request. My wanting to keep certain information private, however, generated a rather lengthy and uncomfortable discussion when I arrived at the office.

When you go to a doctor for the first time, you will usually be asked to sign a form verifying that you have been shown the office's notice of privacy practices and had a chance to review it. Some receptionists had not shown me the privacy information, but they still gave me the form to sign saying that I had read it.

I usually authorize all of my doctors to receive my records. I think it's important that each doctor is aware of all of my medical conditions and treatments. On a rare occasion, as in the case of the dentist, I do not want my records to be shared.

Bring a Flashlight!

Come prepared for emergencies, such as a bathroom with no toilet paper or the lights going out.

You sometimes run into the most bizarre situations at facilities. On two occasions, I was in the bathroom when the lights went out. I now carry a very small flashlight in my pocketbook. I always carry toilet paper in my purse. I also bring water in case the water cooler is empty. Occasionally an office does not have soap, so I also carry a hand sanitizer.

❦❦❦❦

The Waiting Room

The Waiting Room

Don't assume that the order in which patients walk in is the order in which they will be seen.

A lot of things happen in waiting rooms. It's common for one patient to ask another patient what time their appointment is and with which doctor. Patients ask that to find out how long another patient has been waiting and to be sure a person with a later time is not being seen before them.

Some offices take people in the order they arrive, and not according to their scheduled times. Other offices take patients as scheduled, which I think is fair. Someone might be called in first if an x-ray or other test must be taken. If I arrive early, I politely say that I realize I'm early. I don't expect to be taken before others who had appointments ahead of mine.

Consider talking with other patients who want to chat. Otherwise, respect their desire to keep to themselves.

When an office is busy, patients often chat with each other in the waiting room. Three other patients and I once discovered that we all had a two o'clock appointment with the same doctor. One of the patients asked the receptionist why all four of us were scheduled for the same time. She said this allows them to fill all the slots in case someone cancels. Since we all showed up, we were left wondering how the doctor would have time to give each of us a productive visit. It also meant an extremely long wait.

Sometimes you can have rewarding conversations with other patients. It's not uncommon for patients to share their medical journeys with each other. This can be very comforting. Other times, you can sense if a person wants to be alone. Some people don't want to chat and would rather sit and read. You need to respect their privacy.

I've been in some waiting rooms where patients really bonded. I recall a situation in which many of us had been waiting several hours to be called in to the doctor. We applauded each lucky person who finally got called in. That type of bonding helps you deal with the stress of waiting. Sometimes, though, after you get called in for your visit, you are taken to another waiting room to wait some more!

Carry food and water.

You might find yourself getting hungry if you have to wait a long time. I always carry food and water, although some offices don't allow patients to eat or drink in the waiting area or examining room. If I'm very hungry, I'll ask the staff approximately how much longer my wait might be. If it will be a while, I tell the staff I'm stepping out of the office a few minutes to snack. If you have medical problems, such as diabetes or hypoglycemia, you should inform the staff so they know of your needs. An excessively long time in the waiting room can become an emergency for patients who must eat or take medicine at a certain time.

Ask for a place to elevate your limb if you need to.

At orthopedic and podiatry offices, I have frequently observed patients who have a cast on and want to raise their leg up. There is usually no place in the office to do so. If an extra chair is available, some patients use that. If you have ever had a broken limb, you can relate to the tremendous fatigue, heaviness, and swelling that can arise without your limb elevated. It would be helpful if there was something for patients to rest their limbs upon while waiting, especially when their doctors have probably told them to keep their limb elevated. I know of some patients who had to sit for several hours until they were seen.

If someone is accompanying you, perhaps they could carry a small sturdy footstool for you to place your foot on. It won't be as effective as elevating it at a higher level, but it could help alleviate some discomfort. Prior to your appointment, ask the office if they allow patients to bring items to elevate their feet. There could be liability concerns if another patient tripped on a footstool and fell.

You could ask the staff if there is an extra room with an examining table where you could lay down. If the workers are very busy, though, your chances of getting a room to wait in will probably be quite slim.

Prior to an independent medical exam for disability, a technician might secretly be watching you.

When I had my disability review for my employer, I expected there would be a person watching me in the waiting room. Sure enough, there was. Later, I requested the office notes. The notes stated that the person observing me noticed that I was not in pain. I was appalled, because someone would not be able to tell the discomfort I was in by looking at me. I was in great distress from my bladder. My fibromyalgia was flaring up, and my husband was helping me fill out the forms. I feel such judgment, especially for invisible ailments, should be illegal. The number of times I got up to go to the bathroom was also being tracked. My getting up was the only thing they could actually see. The tracking seemed unfair, since my frequency of needing a bathroom can vary by the hour. If I was having excessive urinary frequency, they might think I'm faking it. If I was having a rather good day in terms of frequency, they may not believe that I have worse days.

Videos – No Popcorn

If you don't like the videos, politely inform the staff.

Prior to each chemotherapy session, I had to get a blood test. Each time I sat in the waiting room for my test, the office had videos playing about various types of cancer. It was not uplifting at all. Why would someone who had cancer want to watch videos about other types of cancer? Isn't it enough to deal with the one you have?

I've seen videos at dental offices regarding implants. I find these videos discouraging, and they only make me anxious about my visit. They sometimes seem to be a marketing tool to encourage patients to get a certain procedure done. I realize that the intent may also be educational, but I find them distracting.

Sales Representatives

If you think your visit was rushed to make time for a pharmaceutical representative, tell your doctor.

I cringe when pharmaceutical sales representatives walk into the waiting room with their briefcases of medicines. I know this could mean trouble for my visit from a time perspective. The doctor might see that representative before me or shorten my visit to allow time for the representative. This happened to me at the worst of all times. I had been called to see my doctor to discuss the results of my biopsy. Initially, I was the only one in the waiting room, and I was thinking that at least my visit would not be rushed. Then, in walked a sales representative! I wanted to tell the sales representative to leave, since I was there for a possible cancer diagnosis. The doctor called me in first, but he rushed through the visit. He said he had to cut the visit short in order to meet with the sales representative.

If you think your visit was rushed due to your doctor squeezing in a pharmaceutical representative, tell your doctor. If enough patients speak up about such intrusions, perhaps doctors will find a more efficient way to meet with sales representatives. I don't know if the doctors set up a specific time for them to come in or if they stop in unexpectedly. I also don't know if the sales representatives must speak with a physician or if they can meet with other personnel. I've had occasions in which I saw sales representatives talking to my doctor, and those visits were quite rushed.

Office Magazines, Pens, and Germs

Consider bringing in your own reading material.

One day, while I was reading a magazine in a doctor's office, it occurred to me that there could be a lot of germs on it. Usually, I am not one to think much about germs. After a while, I realized it might be smart to bring my own reading material. Nowadays, many people bring their Kindles or NOOK books. Ask the office what, if any, personal electronic devices are allowed in the office.

When I pick up prescriptions at a pharmacy, I use my pen to initialize forms. Even if a facility does disinfect its pens periodically, it's wise to use your own pen during the flu season.[11] If the person in front of you just used the pen, it won't be disinfected by the time you need to use it.

If you want to bring magazines from the waiting room into the room where the doctor will see you, ask the staff if that's okay.

Did you ever start reading a great article in the waiting room and then suddenly get called in to see the doctor? I once brought a magazine from the waiting room into the examining room. Later, the nurse told me that those magazines were never to be removed from the front waiting room. Some offices might not care. I suggest that you ask the receptionist if magazines from the waiting room are allowed in the treatment rooms.

You might stumble across an article that happens to relate to the very thing for which you are seeing the doctor. You might want to show it to your doctor to get his or her opinion. If that happens, inform the staff person, who will probably say you can bring the magazine into the treatment room.

An office might not want magazines in the treatment room for sanitary reasons. Also, if patients bring magazines into the treatment rooms, there will be fewer magazines available for the waiting area. Magazines also cause clutter in examining rooms.

Chairs

If you think an office's chairs are uncomfortable, politely tell them.

Have you ever wondered why some offices don't have more comfortable chairs in their waiting and treatment rooms? I think a good chair is especially important in orthopedic and physical therapy offices. It also shows that the facility cares about the comfort of its patients. I've experienced wobbly chairs, squishy chairs, and chairs with such a forward tilt that you feel you'll get ejected. Having a good chair for clients just seems like the right thing to do, especially when they may have a long wait. Inform the staff if you think their chairs are uncomfortable.

I am particular about chairs at dental offices. Some treatment chairs are so large and angled that I cannot get comfortable. I don't want to be squirming around during a root canal or dental implant procedure. Some dental hygienists tilt the chairs too far back. I realize they are positioning the chair so that they can work in a more effective manner, but when they almost lay you flat, it can be difficult for those with strong gag reflexes, or neck or back problems. Inform the hygienist if you prefer not to go back too far. Some hygienists will make accommodations for you.

Some offices need more chairs in treatment rooms. If you bring someone to the visit with you, you certainly want that person to have a comfortable place to sit. If you are in need of an extra chair, inform the nurse. If another chair is available, the nurse will usually bring it into the room for you.

Needing a Bathroom

Let the front desk know when you are stepping out to use a restroom.

One thing that can be awkward for a patient is being in a waiting room and suddenly having to use the bathroom. You wonder if the nurse is going to call your name to come into the treatment room while you are in the bathroom. I usually tell the receptionist that I'll be gone for just a few minutes while I use their restroom. Once, I did not do that, and the nurse called my name while I was gone. She thought I had left the office and called the next patient in.

Some places have better bathrooms than others. One office I go to has a bathroom the size of a small closet.

The Nurse Calls You In

How Are You?

Be careful how you answer.

I find it perplexing when nurses ask me how I am. I am not certain if they mean it in a general way, as they would ask anyone, or if they mean it in regards to my illness. If patients reply that they are fine, might the nurse take that to mean that the patients' medical problems no longer bother them? Sometimes people say they are fine to be cordial, even though they are not fine. If you are not on disability, this issue is not a big deal. When you are on disability and constantly put on the defense, however, you have to be concerned with how your comments and appearance are interpreted. I now respond by telling nurses that I'm doing okay except for my feet, back, and bladder.

Don't Look Too Good at Your Appointment

If you have an invisible illness, you might need to speak up to have a medical professional understand the severity of your symptoms.

Perhaps you have an invisible impairment that is disabling to you. If you dress up too nicely, a doctor or nurse might perceive you as being better than you truly are. Several nurses commented on how great I looked upon greeting me. Although I knew they meant well, I found it frustrating because so many of my ailments are invisible. Sometimes I had not slept the night before due to frequent urination, but the nurses didn't notice how tired I was. At one visit, I had severe discomfort in my back, but no one could see my distress as I was standing there. One nurse said that I was lucky that my ailments are invisible. I know she thought she was being kind. The invisible nature of the conditions, however, is what makes them so hard to deal with. People often don't believe what they can't see.

I put blush on one morning prior to an appointment. I asked the doctor for an iron test because he had previously suggested that I get one. He told me that my cheeks were nice and rosy and thus determined that I did not need the test. I told him that my rosy cheeks were due to the blush, but he dismissed it. If you are telling a doctor how tired you are, the doctor may wonder how you had the energy to put on make-up and earrings. If you look too good, the doctor may not believe the severity of your symptoms. Many people look good in their coffin. Obviously, looking good does not always mean that you feel good!

My mother had dementia. Even some of the specialists who treated her thought her condition better than it was because she looked so good.

Blood Pressure Cuff Sizes

If you suspect that the nurse is taking your pressure incorrectly, discuss that with your doctor.

Several years ago, I learned that there are different sizes of blood pressure cuffs. If a cuff is too large for your arm size it can give a false low reading. If it's too small for your arm, it can give a false high reading. I became aware of this when my employer sponsored a day of free blood pressure screenings. I went to have my pressure taken before I ate lunch. The nurse informed me that my arm was too thin for the cuff size that she had. She said she would not take the reading because it's critical that the right size cuff be used for a patient's arm size to obtain an accurate reading.

The next time I went to a doctor, which happened to be at a specialist's office, I bought this subject up. This particular doctor was quite mad at me for bringing it up. She treated me as if she thought I was trying to be a doctor. I was merely asking her what the nurse had instructed me to do. I suspect the issue was that the doctor didn't have more than one cuff size and didn't want patients to know that.

I later found other physicians who understood the importance of the proper cuff size. I once had a doctor that was fantastic in this regard. She even took the time to hunt around the building for the proper cuff for my arm, but she couldn't find it. She took my blood pressure anyway, but she told me that I should get it checked soon with the proper cuff size. I respected her concern and attention to detail.

To get an accurate reading, it is critical that not only a proper cuff size be used for your limb, but also that the cuff be applied to your limb correctly. You want to be relaxed when your pressure is taken. Ask the nurse to be sure your arm is at the correct level to allow for an accurate reading. While sitting down, my understanding is that your elbow should be about at your heart level, your legs should not be dangling, and you should not have had coffee or smoked within a certain time period of the reading[12]. Ask your doctors for specifics and what they think is the proper way for your pressure to be taken. Some nurses have taken my pressure with little regard for the location of my arm. I've had chatty nurses that engage me in discussions while taking my blood pressure. I don't appreciate that, because talking while having your reading taken can elevate your blood pressure. You have to hope that the office is adequately maintaining its blood pressure equipment. One has to wonder how many people might have been put on medication needlessly due to inaccurate readings or faulty equipment. In some patients, with certain conditions, a doctor or nurse might even take your blood pressure while you are standing.[13]

When a person in training takes my blood pressure, I always wonder if they know how to do it accurately. Once, I was at an emergency room in New Jersey. The nurse asked *me* what a normal blood pressure should be. She told me she was a new employee at the facility and could not remember what numbers represented a normal blood pressure reading.

If your blood pressure reads a bit high, ask your doctor if he or she can take more readings another time. Sometimes the pressure can be a bit higher just from the anxiety of sitting in a doctor's office. If it's high, ask your doctor to take a reading in your other arm too. There may be slight variations in the readings between your left and right arm. You don't want to be put on high blood pressure medicines unnecessarily. If the reading was extremely high, however, you would want to take immediate precautions. Discuss such concerns with your doctor to be sure you are not jumping into high blood pressure medicine unnecessarily. Sometimes numerous readings at different times must be taken to fully and accurately assess the need for medication. To help in the overall assessment, your doctor might also suggest that you buy a good quality blood pressure kit to track readings at home. Be sure the kit includes the proper cuff size for your arm.

Discuss your diet, level of physical activity, and medications with your doctor. Salt, natural licorice and other foods may affect your blood pressure. Ask your doctor to try the least invasive means to normalize your blood pressure.

Needing a Bathroom While in a Treatment Room

If you require the frequent use of a bathroom, inform the nurse before the doctor enters the examining room.

Having to use the bathroom is especially troublesome if you are in an examining room prior to the doctor coming in. Once, while waiting for a doctor, I left the treatment room to use the bathroom. When I returned, I was told that the doctor went on to the next patient since I was not there. I had tried to find the nurse to tell her I was temporarily leaving the room but was unable to locate her. That resulted in me having to wait until the doctor was finished with the other patient. By that time, I had to use the bathroom yet again.

It's awkward if you are at the gynecologist's office with a gown on and you have to urinate. Do you whip on your clothes and hope the doctor does not come in just at that moment? Do you run down the hall with your sheet or gown on? I usually opt to run down the hall in my gown.

One time, while at an orthopedic visit, I was told that the bathroom they wanted me to use was upstairs. So, I ended up on the elevator in my gown. The need to use a restroom is especially problematic in offices whose bathroom is in the hallway. The situation is even worse when you need a key for the bathroom.

Gowns

If you can't differentiate the front from the back of a gown, ask.

I laugh when a nurse tells me to put on a gown. I think of the word gown as meaning a fancy evening gown. I'm always in trouble with the one-size-fits-all gowns because I'm very tiny and swim in them. Don't you hate having to figure out how the ties go and if they want the opening in the front or the back? Some gowns have lost their ties, or the Velcro does not stick.

I recently heard about a company that is making more attractive hospital gowns.[14] Finally, some style for patients. Encourage hospitals to purchase more attractive gowns in a wider variety of sizes. I read about a woman who made unique gowns for sick children at a hospital in her area, and it helped to give the children a positive attitude.[15]

I used to think that the length of all gowns came to slightly above or below a patient's knees. A nurse handed me a gown, and I thought she said to take my pants and top off. She left the room while I undressed. I put on the gown while sitting down. As I was getting up from the chair, I noticed that the gown ended slightly above my waistline. At my moment of realization, the nurse happened to walk in, and we both laughed. I sure looked silly, so she told me to put my pants back on. After all these years, I finally learned about the different length gowns.

Unusual Needs

If you have unusual needs, inform your doctor.

Due to foot surgeries that I had several years ago, my feet are very uncomfortable with socks on if I'm also wearing my shoes. Therefore, I will wear socks, and not shoes, when being examined by a dentist or doctor. Nurses and dental hygienists have asked me why I don't have my shoes on. Even after I explain why, they usually tell me to put my shoes on due to liability issues if I fall. This results in my having to ask each practitioner if they would allow me to remove my shoes.

If you have similar issues, discuss them with your practitioners. If they agree to accommodate your needs, inform the hygienists or nurses so they won't have to be concerned.

Keep Your Feet in the Stirrups!

If something seems ridiculous, it might be.

Once, when I was on the table at the gynecologist for a routine exam, the nurse said I must keep my feet in the stirrups until the doctor comes in. After ten minutes of being on the table like that, I realized how silly it was. I took my feet out of the stirrups and sat up. Why couldn't I just put my feet up once the doctor was in the room? Furthermore, isn't it a bit strange to have a doctor walk in and greet you while your legs are wide open? It only takes a few seconds for a patient to put their feet in the stirrups. When the nurse came in with the doctor, she was not happy that I had moved. It's possible the doctor had requested she use that procedure. Either way, the whole thing seemed silly to me.

If a nurse asks you to do something that seems silly, ask why you must do that. You can then discuss the necessity further with the nurse. A nurse or technician might have very good reasons for telling you to keep still. You certainly do not want to move after being positioned for an x-ray.

Thick Patient Files

Be aware of the pitfalls of a thick patient file.

If you frequent your doctor a lot, your file might become quite thick. A fat file can work against you in many ways. The doctor might think you are coming in too much, that you are compulsive, or that you are taking advantage of the disability system.

That's unfair if you are truly trying to get help and searching for a treatment or cure.

The files that my doctors have on me have become very thick. I often saw my doctors hunting around in them for information. Sometimes my doctors gave up trying to find something. One of my doctors could not find my list of allergies. I later mailed him an updated list of my allergies and requested that it be kept in a visible place in my file.

Although the use of electronic medical records will eliminate thick files, it still won't prevent a patient's lengthy medical history from showing in a computer system.

Multiple Allergies

Accurately describe your reactions to medications.

During your initial appointment, you will be asked to inform the office of any medicines to which you are allergic or have had adverse reactions. When I tell doctors or nurses that I am allergic to four medications, they usually look at me in disbelief. Some laughed at me and treated me as if I was strange because I was allergic to so many medications.

I never understood why someone would be surprised that a person reacts to more than a few medications. Medications are not natural to the body. If you think about it, doesn't it make more sense that a person could have an adverse reaction to medications? Instead of laughing at the patient, I think a practitioner should applaud the patient for keeping track of reactions and informing the doctor about them.

Accurately describe your reactions to medications. Then, your doctor can determine which medicine(s) truly caused an allergic reaction. Hives would indicate an allergic reaction, but feeling a bit of nausea might just be a negative side effect.

Excessive Tests

If you think an x-ray is not necessary, tell the nurse you'd like to discuss the necessity of it with your doctor.

On one occasion, I made an appointment for a consultation with my doctor. After the nurse called me in, she started to walk me to the x-ray machine. I told her I did not need or want x-rays because I was there for a consultation, not an examination. Furthermore, the doctor had recently examined my x-ray results. The nurse was taken aback, but after talking to the doctor, she agreed x-rays were not needed.

If you think that testing is being done unnecessarily, talk to your doctor about your concern. Your doctor might have a valid reason for ordering certain tests. On the other hand, sometimes tests are given merely as a routine and are not needed.

High Examining Tables

If you need help getting on and off an examination table, inform the nurse and doctor.

Have you ever been cranked up so high at a podiatrist's office that you thought you'd hit the ceiling? I was in quite a dilemma the first time this happened to me. I didn't expect anyone would raise me that high. By the time I realized that I had to go to the bathroom, the nurse had already left the room. No one was around, so I had to jump a few feet to the ground. It would be better if the chair were only raised once the doctor comes into the room. Even going up a foot or so can be treacherous for a frail person.

If you think that you have been raised too high, inform the staff. They may not realize that you might need to get off of the examining chair or table while waiting for the doctor to come into the room.

Most doctors have a table that is not too high, but might still require a patient to jump up to get on it. A stepstool is usually nearby, but not always. Getting up on tables can be especially difficult if a patient has an injury. I remember my parents telling me they had concerns about getting on and off examining tables. They were afraid they'd end up with more problems than they already had if they fell. I wish all offices had an examining table that a doctor could raise or lower as needed for each patient. I have only seen them in a few offices.

Closed Doors

If you prefer to have the examining room door open while waiting for your doctor, ask the staff person who brought you to the room if they would keep it open if you don't have to undress while waiting.

I hate sitting for a long time in an examining room when the door is shut, assuming I'm fully dressed. I feel closed in and rather lonely. I usually open the door to let air in. I can hear the nurses and doctors as they go up and down the hallway. If I hear my doctor walk into another examining room, I know it's a good time for me to use the bathroom, if I need to. It also gives me an idea how much longer I may have to wait. I've always wondered if doctors mind that I open the door. Perhaps a closed door is a signal that a patient is waiting in the room. Of course, the staff obviously closes doors for privacy reasons.

❦❦❦❦

The Visit with Your Doctor

Bring an Advocate to Your Appointment

Bring someone to your visit to take notes, be an observer, and ask questions for you if you are not able to ask questions yourself.

It's helpful to have an advocate with you if you are discussing an upcoming procedure or surgery. You can ask your advocate to take notes during the visit. If legally allowed, some patients bring a recording device to record the visit. Your doctor, however, may find recording a bit intrusive. Much depends on the nature of the visit and your doctor's attitude.

Try to bring an advocate who is not talkative. If he or she gets too chatty with the doctor, it steals time from your visit, and time is precious. Your advocate should be there primarily as a listener, unless you need him or her to ask questions that you may not physically or mentally be able to. It's best to bring someone who is not overwhelmed by medical lingo and who can handle some of the queasy stuff. Prior to your visit, talk to your advocate about what you expect his or her role to be. In some situations, doctors can ask advocates to leave if they feel the advocate's presence is interfering with your care.

There is a great need for health-care advocates to accompany patients to their visits. If you are lucky, you have friends and family members who live locally and have the experience to be a proficient advocate. Some patients, unfortunately, do not have such contacts. Our society needs paid staff or volunteers who are trained as health-care advocates for patients who desire one. Having someone with you at visits should be the norm, not an exception.

How Many Questions Can You Ask at a Visit?

Bring a list of questions with you to your visit.

It's helpful to make a list of what you want to discuss with your doctor and bring it to your appointment. Keep your questions brief and to the point, and don't ramble. I've read articles in which patients were advised to bring a lengthy list of questions to their doctor. The reality is that there will not be enough time at a typical office visit for too many questions. Asking numerous questions can make a doctor think that you don't want the treatment or that you may present a legal problem if something goes wrong. Some doctors will be more willing than others to answer questions. If you feel your questions aren't adequately answered, or you do not understand the doctor's response, tell your doctor. Some of my doctors were very good about answering questions. One doctor, however, told me that I asked too many questions. He actually took my notes from me and tossed them in the garbage. My questions were about an upcoming surgery and were very important to me. He told me I was unusual and overly concerned. I was frustrated by his reaction, because I knew I was being a smart patient who was not getting the respect I deserved.

If you have a long list of questions, start your visit with the ones that are most important to you. At the beginning of your visit, tell your doctor that getting an answer to all of your questions is important to you. I usually tell my doctors that I realize they may not have time to answer all of my questions during one visit, and then I inform them that I'll follow up shortly during another visit. Sometimes I set up two appointments not too far apart to allow me to get all the answers I need. Some receptionists discouraged me from setting up two appointments, but I insisted, because I knew that all of my questions would not be answered during one visit.

Some clerical questions can be answered by a nurse or doctor's assistant. Such questions might cover such things as where to buy a specific product the doctor suggested or what days the doctor performs surgery. Be cautious about staff members who act as if they can answer more than they are trained to handle. I've found that some nurses and staff members are overly protective of a doctor's time and try to answer questions that only a doctor should answer. I called a doctor's office once and asked if the doctor would call me back regarding a question I had. The receptionist who answered the phone transferred me to a woman who she thought could answer my question. I wanted to know if it was okay that I get a certain treatment. She responded, "I don't see why not, since it can't hurt you."

I later found out that a person should not have more than twelve of those treatments in a year. The woman I spoke with did not ask me if I had undergone those treatments before. She also did not take into account that I may need more of those treatments later in the year. She should have asked the doctor my question or allowed me to schedule an appointment with him.

Sometimes you might think your question will take only a moment to answer. The doctor may know that the answer is more involved than you thought, which can result in your doctor having to get more information from you before you move on to the next question. You have to be flexible, since the doctor is trying to help you. If the doctor needs time to also examine x-rays, it will cut into your discussion time. I'm not discouraging you from bringing in x-rays. Be aware, however, that it will steal some time for other concerns.

I think a full hour is often needed to discuss an upcoming surgery. The doctor needs time to answer your questions and perhaps to examine you further and tell you his or her treatment plan. You might need to ask the doctor what supplies you'll need when you get home and how often you have to come into the office in the weeks following the surgery. These details all take time to discuss. Good luck finding a doctor who will give you a full hour, though. I usually book two half-hour visits ahead of time to allow for such discussions.

We Have Time to Discuss Only Two Issues

If the office has a sign telling you to discuss no more than two body parts during a visit, don't always take it literally.

I've seen signs at offices that say a patient should discuss only two body parts during one visit. The insurance company may have limited the amount of time that a doctor can spend with each patient. The limitation of two body parts is not in the best interest of the patient and may be detrimental in assessing what is wrong. Fifteen minutes may not be enough time to assess a patient thoroughly for certain afflictions.

Suppose you tell your doctor that your hips and back hurt. If you see a sign telling you to discuss no more than two body parts, you might be afraid to tell your doctor that your feet also hurt. It's a shame that patients can't feel free to tell their doctors about their other ailments. All three of those discomforts could be related. They could also signal that additional x-rays are needed to help in a diagnosis.

One of my doctors told me that I should bring up only one or two topics at a visit. She said that my mentioning all of my discomforts would be confusing to a doctor. In my case, many of my discomforts are related to my overall problem of fibromyalgia. My complaints might seem like different issues to a doctor making a quick assessment, but many of my discomforts are related to one condition.

If you think that more than two issues might be related to your overall problem, inform your doctor despite any sign hanging up. Your doctor can then assess how much focus should be spent on your other issue(s). My guess is the doctor will be understanding and realize the significance of what you are saying.

Do You Mind if an Intern Watches?

Speak up and be honest as to whether or not you want an intern to sit in on your visit.

I used to allow medical students to sit in on my office visits. I knew the interns needed to learn, and often the doctor spent more time with me, which I liked. On the other hand, sometimes it was disruptive to my care. One day, I was looking forward to talking to my practitioner about some private medical issues. That was the one time that she asked if someone could sit in on my visit. I timidly said yes, and I regretted it for a long time. Over the years, I've learned to say no. It's a bit awkward saying no in front of the person in training, but you need to do what's best for you. The practitioner should ask patients how they feel about it, prior to bringing the person in training into the room, which would eliminate some of the awkwardness. Otherwise, it puts pressure on patients to say yes, when they might want to say no.

Do You Mind if Another Doctor Sees You Today?

While in an examining room, you may be asked if another physician can see you instead of your own physician. Speak up if you want to wait and see your own doctor.

Don't be surprised if occasionally you are asked if it's okay if another doctor sees you instead of your own doctor. That happened to me a few times during my office visits for ovarian cancer. It surprised me, because when I had made the appointments, I emphasized that I wanted to see only my doctor. Upon my entrance into the examining room, an assistant encouraged me to change my mind. I stood my ground and waited because my doctor was one of the top doctors in the country. I was not going to see just anyone, when my life was on the line. I realize there may be a situation when your own doctor really cannot see you. I found this situation to happen mostly at teaching hospitals with clinics. My intent is not to show disrespect for teaching hospitals, since they often provide excellent care for patients, but sometimes your wait can be longer at teaching hospitals.

What's the Diagnosis?

Don't give up on getting a proper diagnosis.

One of your challenges as a patient is getting the proper diagnosis. If you have an uncommon illness, or one that your doctor is not familiar with, you may have to see several doctors in various locations before you get a diagnosis. If your doctor can't find anything objectively wrong, friends and family may assume you are okay. Perhaps there is no test developed yet to detect what you have, or perhaps you haven't been given the correct test. Those close to you may not believe how much you are suffering if you have invisible symptoms. You know the pain is real and that you deserve more understanding than you may be getting.

If you have an illness that your doctor says there is no cure or treatment for, it's important that you challenge that viewpoint. You might be surprised what may surface from your own research. If you can't do your own research, ask a family member or friend to help. Some libraries will perform a limited amount of research for you, sometimes for a fee. There is a wealth of information online, but be sure to use reputable sites. You can ask librarians, patient advocacy groups, and your doctors if they know of reputable sites. Some of my doctors frowned upon my research, yet others applauded my efforts and determination. Share the results of your research with a doctor to get his or her professional opinion of it.

Support groups can be helpful and can usually put you in touch with national organizations that can provide further information. They may know of treatments that your doctor is not aware of. You can then discuss the pros and cons of those treatments with your doctor. Sometimes just talking with others who share similar experiences can be motivating and enlightening.

If you have a condition for which it is difficult to get a diagnosis, you may have to see several specialists. Be aware, however, that you might then end up with multiple diagnoses. I've had different doctors diagnose the same issue differently. It makes you question just who, if anyone, is correct.

In 1992, I had some type of attack in my left foot. It felt as if the nerve were being zapped, and it resulted in my suddenly having very uncomfortable sensations in my foot and leg. I had just walked five miles prior to the attack, and after it, I could barely walk across the room. A neurosurgeon thought I would no longer be walking or speaking by the end of the year. A neurologist thought I might have multiple sclerosis. Orthopedics thought it was from my back. Osteopaths thought it was a soft tissue problem. I had my own theory. You can see how easily a person with an unusual condition can end up with multiple diagnoses. Each specialist will probably see things from his or her own perspective.

Don't accept that nothing can be done for you. Don't give up!

Do You Remember Me?

Don't assume that your doctor will remember every detail of your medical history.

Do you ever feel like your doctor does not remember your case from one visit to the next? Keep in mind that doctors see numerous patients, and it is probably difficult for them to recall the details of each case, especially if the patient does not come to the office frequently. You need to take some responsibility for keeping your doctor abreast of your issues. One time, I was given a medication that I was told must be monitored every four to six weeks. Upon researching the medication, I decided not to take it. To my surprise, the doctor did not bring up the issue until nearly a year later, even though I had been in the office a few times in between.

I was surprised that one of my practitioners, who had seen me occasionally over the last few years, acted as if he had not seen me for thirty years. He even welcomed me back to his office. I saved him the embarrassment by keeping silent instead of telling him that he had treated me just a few years before. I think doctors are so busy these days that they don't have time to go through their patient files thoroughly.

I cannot stress enough the importance of keeping your doctors abreast of your issues. If you don't, a doctor may end up repeating tests, ignoring important matters, or taking you down the wrong road. Being too polite to avoid confrontations may cost you in terms of getting the proper treatment.

Conversational Styles

Be aware of conversational styles and how much they affect the communication between you and your doctor.

I appreciate a doctor who, at the beginning of a visit, asks patients why they are there. Some doctors begin discussing treatments before patients even had a chance to tell them why they set up the appointment, which can throw things off track. When that happens, I tell the doctors that I'll be glad to return to their issues, but that I came in to discuss something else. This tactic lets the doctor know that time is needed to address your topics in addition to their own. It would be helpful if the structure and purpose of each visit were established upfront; unfortunately, there is not a lot of time during a visit to allow for agendas.

Sometimes a manner of speaking can throw off a visit. One doctor almost kicked me out of the room when I used a technical word. I was familiar with the word because I frequently came across medical terminology while writing insurance contracts at work. He said I was using too big a word, and he perceived me as trying to diagnose myself. He was making a quick and unfair assessment of me.

A doctor's tone of voice has a lot to do with how seriously I take his or her advice. One of my doctors, who is rather soft spoken, politely told me that he had a concern with the scar tissue that may come from the foot surgery I was contemplating. His comment did not sound important to me. I was used to my father's voice, which was much louder and firmer if something was truly important. It's interesting how our upbringing can affect how we respond to a doctor's comments.

I also appreciate a doctor who is efficient in answering questions and does not go off on unnecessary tangents. One of my surgeons loves to draw pictures about what he is explaining. I felt that the drawings took precious time away from the important questions I still had. Many times I left his office feeling frustrated. I realize the doctor was trying to help me. Some people are naturally inclined to express themselves by using diagrams and drawings. I prefer a verbal approach, rather than pictorial. If you visit a certain doctor frequently and find that his or her drawings are getting in the way of your discussion time, politely tell your doctor that you grasp things better when they are conveyed verbally to you.

Don't we all appreciate a doctor who is a good listener? It's equally important that patients listen intently to their doctors' advice. I also respect doctors whose body language reflects that they are taking in what you are saying. A keen listener will make good eye contact and not be distracted by looking around the room or nodding out. If doctors type into a computer while with you, it does not seem like they are fully listening to you.

I also appreciate a doctor who talks to me while I am fully dressed, not just when I am on the examining table wearing a paper sheet. It's intimidating to have a conversation with a doctor while you are sitting half naked on a table.

Some of my doctors have asked me to put on a gown while they leave the room. Most of them return rather quickly. Once, however, a doctor told me to put on a gown and said he'd return in a few minutes. It was around noontime when he said that. After about thirty minutes of waiting, I had to go to the bathroom. I got dressed and went down the hallway to inquire where the bathroom was. I overheard several people laughing and talking in an area at the far end of the hallway. The doctor was in there with his staff eating lunch. He did not come back to the treatment room until one o'clock. It was obvious to me that when he told me to put on the gown, he knew he'd be spending nearly a full hour down the hall eating lunch. I thought it was very rude of him to leave me sitting on the table with a gown on for so long. Why couldn't he have told me to sit in the waiting room awhile?

Some doctors discuss things from a very logical perspective. One of my doctors bluntly told me that he is a very logical and scientific kind of guy. I appreciated his being upfront about it, especially since my style is quite the opposite. Knowing our different styles enabled us to communicate better.

On occasion, I've come across practitioners whose tone and language borders on abusive. Usually it is their ego getting in the way of treatment. Only once did I have a practitioner actually scream at me. It happened when I mentioned that I might use the services of another practitioner whose office was closer to where I lived. He also told me that he did not respect that practitioner, and he used vulgar language to describe him. His voice grew louder and louder and his face red, as he continued to rant about the other practitioner. It was unprofessional, not to mention that those in the nearby waiting room could hear him. What do you do in a situation like that? Keep calm, and do not yell back. I listened to him and then later politely told the receptionist that I would not be returning to his office. I had seen that practitioner a few times before and had liked and respected him very much. Others had warned me of his outbursts. I believed them, but I had not experienced it until that day.

Be proactive in getting your doctor to pay attention to detail.

I greatly respect and appreciate a practitioner's attention to detail; otherwise, seemingly simple things can go amiss. Some of the practitioners I saw for vision care did not remind me to wear sunglasses outside, after having my eyes dilated. Likewise, some dentists had not suggested that I clean the retainers they made for me. This lack of attention to detail can cause further problems for a patient. The issue of after-care is too important to be dismissed.

Consider how open-minded your doctor is.

I once had a reaction to a particular medication. My doctor insisted that the medicine could have not have caused the problem, even though the manufacturer's flyer said it could. That kind of attitude from a doctor leaves you at a dead end. Numerous patients have told me that their doctors did not take reactions to medications seriously. One of my doctors didn't care that I broke into hives when I took a certain medication, and she told me to continue to take the medicine anyway. I appreciate a doctor who considers what a patient says, even though it may seem odd or unusual. Doctors can learn a lot by listening and being open-minded. Patients are often dismissed as being anxious and overly concerned because they question a medication. Doctors should instead be telling their patients how smart they are to bring medication issues to their doctors' attention.

What Is the Definition of "Better"?

Be careful how you use the word "better" when talking to your doctor.

"Better" is a relative term. Even though you feel a bit better, you can still be in a lot of pain. "Better" does not automatically mean that you feel good. You don't want misinterpretations in the office notes about your health status, especially if you are on disability. I told one of my doctors that my pain was temporarily a bit better, but I also emphasized it was still very bad. The notes, however, said that I was doing better. A disability reviewer could interpret such a statement as the patient being better than he or she actually is. If your doctor makes such a note, ask the doctor to clarify the notes.

Revealing the Names of Other Doctors

Use caution when freely giving out the names of other doctors you have seen.

Soon after I entered an examining room, a doctor told me he thought foot surgery would not be good for me. I wondered if he said it because he didn't have experience with the type of surgery I needed. If that was the case, he should have suggested that I see another doctor who was better equipped to perform the surgery. When I brought up the name of a surgeon who was willing to do the surgery, he said that surgery was a good idea. It left me wondering if he changed his mind because he knew the surgeon was excellent or because he personally knew the surgeon. Sometimes I try to keep names of other doctors confidential for this reason. I am amazed by doctors who change their outlook when a patient brings up the name of another doctor.

I had a similar situation concerning a dental x-ray. A dentist told me that it would be malpractice for a dentist to suggest that a certain tooth of mine be extracted. When I told him the name of the dentist who said to pull it, he changed his mind and said that it would be okay to pull it. He told me he had a great deal of respect for that dentist and to trust his expertise. A quick change of opinion by a doctor can leave a patient wondering what is appropriate for their situation.

On one occasion, I was glad I had informed my doctor of another surgeon I was seeing. In that event, my doctor warned me not to go to that practitioner for good reasons. You have to examine the entire situation when deciding how much you want to reveal to your doctor about the names of other specialists you have seen or want to see.

Discussing Surgery with Your Doctor

If a surgical procedure is not urgent, ask your doctor his or her opinion of the surgery, not just during one office visit, but also a few months later.

If you are considering a surgical procedure that is not of an urgent nature, it's helpful to go back to your surgeon again to see if he or she still has the same opinion. I asked a surgeon about a certain procedure. During my first visit, he said the procedure was a great option for me, and he highly recommended it. When I asked him about it a few months later, even though my status had not changed, he suddenly thought it was not a good idea. One could argue that in the meantime he had discovered something negative about the procedure. I think the more likely scenario was that he didn't recall what he had told me the first time or that he had not initially taken the time to assess if I truly was a good candidate for surgery. Hasty office visits can lead a patient down the wrong path. Ask your doctors how often they have performed the surgery you need and how successful those surgeries were.

Sometimes, it is not to your advantage to delay a surgery. I put off a surgery for nearly a year. When I finally called the office to be put on their surgical list, the receptionist told me my doctor was leaving the practice.

Who Is the Back-Up Doctor?

Find out what doctor will take over in the event something happens to your doctor.

Have you thought about what doctor would treat you if your doctor were not available? Knowing your doctor's substitute is especially important in surgical situations. I like to have an idea of who may be stepping in. Ideally, you want to have confidence in any doctor who could be filling in for your regular doctor.

It's good to bring this subject up at your first visit. You can politely ask your regular doctor which doctor would take over for him or her. My husband had a fantastic orthopedic doctor who was suddenly out of the office for an extended time. Fortunately, my husband respected and liked the other doctor who took over his care.

When Doctors Shift Responsibility

Speak up if you believe that your practitioners are unfairly shifting their responsibility.

Years ago, my doctor, who is now deceased, diagnosed me with ovarian cancer. He sent me to a facility outside of my local geographic area to have the surgery so that one of the most skilled physicians in our country could perform it. I was very happy with the arrangement until the after-care. The surgical doctor wanted the doctor who diagnosed me to take over all aspects of follow-up care. The doctor who diagnosed me, however, said that the surgeon should take over my care. For some reason, neither one wanted to take the responsibility.

Prior to my undergoing chemotherapy that would be administered intravenously, I needed to get approval to be catheterized for the treatments. Because of my bladder condition, interstitial cystitis, I do not have the bladder capacity to hold large amounts of fluid. My doctor said that the facility should initiate the catheterization. The facility said that the doctor should initiate it. I had to get very assertive to get my doctor to send the facility a letter noting that I needed to be catheterized during chemotherapy. The facility seemed concerned with liability in the event that I got a bladder infection. Initially, the facility tried to convince me that I did not need to be catheterized. I insisted on it, because I knew I did. Once the treatments began, the nurse said she could clearly understand why I had to be catheterized. She even complimented me for having spoken up.

Your Doctor's Relative Has the Same Disease as You

If your doctor mentions that his or her family member has the same medical condition that you have, use that information to your advantage.

Sometimes, if you are lucky, your doctor's relative will have the same ailment as you. It happened to me once. The doctor was very understanding, because his wife had the same disease. He even gave me his wife's phone number so that I could discuss various treatment options with her. I felt bad that she too had the same condition, but it was certainly positive from my end to have a doctor who believed and understood what I was going through. Your doctor may even know of support groups in your area for specific medical conditions.

"Just Talking"

You might need to explain to your doctor why you have to "just talk" during a visit, as opposed to seeking a particular treatment or solution.

I noticed that some of my doctor's notes said that I spent most of the time talking during the visit. I don't know if doctors put that information merely as a fact and observation, or because they thought I was wasting their time by not seeking a particular treatment. Some doctors think they are not helping you if they are not giving you a prescription or some form of treatment.

It was important to tell my doctors what activities I could not perform, because such facts would be used in my disability assessment. I never felt that my doctors had time to grasp the full scope of what I was going through. I hear this complaint from other patients over and over again.

I should have informed my doctors, at the beginning of the visit, why my discussion was very critical for disability purposes. I don't think my doctors understood the significance of such details in the notes.

Is Your Doctor Current?

Ask your surgeons if they are trained in the latest technology. Ask doctors how up-to-date their medical equipment is.

Some patients told me that they prefer a doctor who has many years of experience. Others told me that they prefer a young doctor who is more likely to be aware of, and trained in, the latest technology. You have to weigh all the factors and consider what your preferences are. I like the best of both worlds. I want a doctor who is very experienced and who also keeps up with the latest technology. It's sometimes hard to find everything you want in one doctor. Some will be aware of helpful procedures that other practitioners may never have heard of. The latest technology may help you get a diagnosis.

I once brought a set of dental x-rays to another dentist for a second opinion. I was surprised when he told me that the x-rays were of such poor quality that he could not see much from them. This dentist then used a better x-ray machine which took outstanding pictures of my teeth. Those pictures enabled him to give me an accurate diagnosis.

Psychological Onslaught

Challenge doctors who say you have an anxiety disorder if you think the ailment is not psychological.

If you are on disability, don't be surprised if your practitioner asks you how your marriage is and what your spouse does for a living. One might ask these questions even if you are not on disability. When there are few objective findings, doctors may look for psychological causes. At times, it felt like my practitioners wanted me to have a bad marriage. I was asked where my husband worked and what his job was. Sometimes I'd be asked about my childhood. Don't be surprised if you get asked what you do with your spare time. It all felt very intrusive. Over time, those treating me grew to see how honest and truthful I was and backed off from such questions. I realize, on some level, they thought they were helping me. It was very discouraging to me, though, and it only set up a defensive environment which was counterproductive to healing.

Over the years, several patients told me that their doctors said their problems were from psychological causes. Those patients may have truly suffered from something physical that had not yet been identified. Some of them were eventually diagnosed by another physician. Their diagnoses included cancer, endometriosis, ulcers, ectopic pregnancy, hydrocephalus, interstitial cystitis, and multiple sclerosis. I have heard such stories from neighbors, friends, family members, and others of all ages and walks of life. I mean no disrespect for those who are truly suffering from such ailments as depression or anxiety. I believe all illnesses, even those considered psychological, have an underlying physical reason. I think some doctors dismiss ailments as psychological for their own convenience, or because they won't admit that they are unable to diagnose a patient.

Am I on Trial?

It may be helpful to bring a family member or friend to your visit.

When a doctor treats patients as if they are exaggerating the severity of their symptoms, it can be hurtful and humiliating. Sometimes it's difficult for patients to prove how much their pain affects their daily activities, especially if their symptoms are invisible to others and if test results are normal.

Another problem can occur when a doctor asks a patient to walk a few steps across the room so that the doctor can identify the patient's walking impairment. The patient might not exhibit the symptoms in such short strides, and pain might vary from day to day. What a doctor sees within a few minutes may not give a true representation of the patient's problems.

A patient on disability might be viewed as pretending to have impairments to gain disability benefits. This distrust sets up a competitive relationship between a doctor and a patient in which each defends his or her position; it only hinders effective treatment. It's also a time and money waster. The time could be better spent listening to patients, believing them, and finding ways to help them. I realize doctors must be on the lookout for fraudulent patients. Most patients, however, are probably not looking for a free ride.

I always wished that my doctors knew about my prior accomplishments. They would have seen a history of a highly motivated person. Certainly, I would not want to lose my job, income, friends, and possibly family relationships, when I had worked so hard to have a good life.

When you come to your appointment, it will be helpful to bring a friend or relative who has observed your limitations. If your physician realizes that another person has seen what you are describing, it may help you appear more credible to the doctor.

Contradictions

If your doctors contradict themselves, politely ask for clarification.

One of the things I often hear from other patients is that their doctors contradict themselves. I am astounded by the number of times my practitioners have done so. For example, one practitioner suggested I use a particular cream that costs more than twenty-five dollars. At my next visit, being the good patient that I was, I proudly informed the doctor that I had bought the cream. His response was, "Why did you buy that? You don't need it." I spared him the embarrassment and kept silent. I should have reminded him that he had told me to buy it.

Some doctors told me I had a certain disorder, and then a few months later, said I could not possibly have it. It seemed they were just saying things to have some type of response. After such situations, I wondered what was true and what wasn't. Doctors who frequently contradict themselves lose credibility with me.

One of my doctors, with whom I had multiple surgeries over the years, always put stitches in me. I normally set up appointments ahead of time to have the stitches out, because I had to plan rides. At one visit, prior to the surgery, I proudly informed the doctor that I had set up an appointment to have my stitches removed. He said, "Why did you do that? I never put stitches in." My husband was at the appointment with me. We both were shocked, as it was a total contradiction to the fact.

Point out to your doctors any contradictions they make. It may be awkward, but they might even appreciate it. If you don't do so, how will you know which suggestion to follow?

Patients Interrupting Other Patients

Be considerate of other patients' privacy.

Have you ever been in a treatment room when another patient walks in during your visit to talk to your practitioner? Such interruptions are rude, especially when others don't excuse themselves. Patients should be considerate of each other's space and treatment time. Practitioners should close the door, if possible. An open door is too inviting in an area that should be private. If the door is left open and another patient walks in, practitioners should explain that a session is in progress and that they cannot talk at the moment.

Other Interruptions

Be patient with interruptions that are warranted.

Haven't we all had interruptions during a visit with our doctors? You have to be patient, to a certain extent. The doctor may be awaiting an important call, or a nurse may need to knock on the door for a valid reason. I had a visit with a specialist for which phone calls seemed too numerous to be justified. It was my first visit with this doctor, and I was told I'd have at least forty-five minutes with him. I counted eight interruptions during my visit, while the doctor took phone calls from patients in front of me. It is possible the calls were urgent, but it seems unlikely to have that many urgent calls within forty-five minutes.

Have you ever noticed practitioners shouting out across the room to each other about their weekend and other personal issues? That type of behavior does not foster a healing environment. A few times, I was trying to tell the person treating me that something she was doing seemed significant to my case, but the person could not hear me, with all the talking going on in the room.

If you experience too many interruptions during your visit, tell your practitioner. It might make your practitioner realize how disrespectful such distractions are to patients. Perhaps it would encourage the office to set up strict guidelines regarding interruptions. Many patients may act like the interruptions don't bother them, when they really do. There may be times, however, when a patient wants to chat a little bit with someone and does not mind an interruption. We are social creatures, and it's natural to want to connect with others. Just don't let it get in the way of your treatment. Even patients sometimes interrupt their practitioners too much. Don't make the person treating you lose focus because you are too chatty.

When Your Practitioner is Too Concerned with Costs

If costs are not a factor for you, tell your practitioner. It may open up more treatment options for you.

The person treating you might try too hard to cut costs for you. By doing so, you could miss out on treatments you would have liked to try. You may be in a situation where money is not of great concern to you. Everyone's financial situation is different. You may think a certain piece of medical equipment is worth the cost to you because of how much it might help you. It could also save you money in the long run, if it does help you.

I usually get two or three custom-made orthotics every two years. The convenience of having multiple orthotics works for me, despite the cost. My orthotics last longer, because moving orthotics from one shoe to another wears out the orthotics faster, if they have a soft material over the top like mine do.

Does Your Practitioner Use New Treatments?

Be honest with your practitioner about how your treatment is going.

You may be receiving physical therapy, massage, or another treatment with which you are very happy. Your practitioner then might want to try a new technique, which can be beneficial in some ways. You could be helped by something that you never would have known about unless you tried it. On the other hand, sometimes staying with the same treatment is the best for the patient. The patient may not need the latest fad or technique. Speak up, if you prefer to continue with your usual treatment. Tell your practitioner how you feel about it, and ask why a new method is being used. Your practitioner might have a very good reason for using certain techniques.

Your practitioner may want to try a new piece of equipment on you. Ask your practitioner about the pros and cons of the product. If your practitioner has not tried it out on many other people, do you really want to be the first one to do so? I prefer to wait until such treatments are proven to be effective and until my practitioner has a lot of experience with the equipment.

Will Your Practitioner Back You Up?

Tell your practitioners if you receive poor service from companies they use.

If you received poor service, or a product of poor quality from a company that your practitioner uses, you probably think that your practitioner will back you up and call the company. My experience is that few practitioners do that. Most likely they don't want to threaten their relationship with the company, or they don't want to take the time. Some may even ask you to make the call, which usually is not productive, since many companies will talk directly only with practitioners. If your practitioner won't help you, you may need to seek out another practitioner. I respect practitioners who demand high-quality service from the companies they deal with. It shows a respect for their patients and upholds good customer service, as well.

You could also run into a similar problem with a disability situation. Your practitioners may have told you, on numerous occasions, that they understand your hardships and limitations. If there is no test to substantiate what you have, however, your practitioner might be reluctant to write a letter for disability purposes that states such limitations. Keep notes on all conversations that you have with practitioners. If you have very good notes and can back yourself up, then your practitioner may be more likely to back you up.

How Often Should You See Your Doctor?

Work out an agreeable schedule with your doctor for the frequency of your visits.

Usually, as doctors are leaving the treatment room after seeing you, they will tell you when you should come in again, if continued care is needed. Sometimes a doctor might say you need to come in only one or two times a year. If you are on disability, the disability reviewers may want you to see the doctor more frequently. From the patient's viewpoint, it can be very helpful to have extra appointments set up. I find it useful to book multiple appointments in case a new treatment comes up that I was not aware of, or in case the doctor has to reschedule me. It shows the disability reviewers that you are being proactive in your care and trying to get better.

It's also good to have an extra appointment in place to allow for disability paperwork that might suddenly arise. If you wait until the last minute, it's often hard to get an appointment as soon as you need it. Usually disability reviewers have to receive paperwork back within a certain timeframe. You will need time to see the doctor, to have the doctor complete the paperwork, and to send the paperwork to the reviewer. If the doctor's letter has errors in it, you will need an appointment to go over the mistakes with the doctor.

Having appointments in place is also critical when it comes to appeal letters and letters for attorneys. An appeal letter that is sent too late can result in your losing an appeal. I was shocked at the amount of critical grammatical errors in some of my physicians' letters. Not only is it embarrassing to send out a letter with grammatical errors, but it also does not look credible. You may have a fantastic doctor, but the doctor or medical clerk may not have the skills to write a good letter. Some doctors interpreted my extra appointments as compulsive, whereas I was just being a smart patient who had to manage various aspects of my care.

If you have a chronic condition, take a few minutes during your office visit to discuss how frequently your doctor wants to see you. If you think you need more visits than your doctor suggests, explain your logic to your doctor.

Some doctors don't realize how strict the disability review guidelines are, in terms of the number of visits a patient needs. My employer originally wanted me to touch base with my doctor every month, but my doctor thought that schedule was too frequent. If you don't explain your reasons for frequent visits, your doctor might view you as overly concerned.

The Specialist in Your Doctor's Office

Don't assume that it's best to see the specialist that comes into your doctor's office.

Your doctors may suggest you see a specialist that comes into their office. It's convenient, and most people have faith that their doctor has selected a good practitioner. I think such specialists are not as available as they would be if you went to them on your own. I have also sensed that some were wary of overstepping the authority of my own practitioner. If you have a bad relationship with the specialists, it can affect the relationship with your own doctor. I prefer to go to all specialists outside of my own doctor's office. You'll have to weigh the pros and cons and see what works best for you.

I had been seeing one of my practitioners for nearly thirty years and was very happy with his services. One day he suggested that I see a specialist who came into his office. I was very pleased with the first exam I had with this specialist; yet after a few visits, something went amiss with the communication. My regular practitioner apologized and said that he had caused part of the mishap. The mishap resulted in my having to get my procedure done elsewhere, because his specialist no longer wanted to treat me. The time wasted cost me thousands of dollars, because additional treatments had to be done, since so much time elapsed. To this day, my relationship with my regular practitioner is not the same. I sense the tension when I walk in the office.

Be Careful Who You Complain To

Use caution when complaining about a staff member. Some staff members are related.

There may be times when you think a receptionist is rude or incompetent. I once spoke to my doctor about a staff member of his that was repeatedly rude to me. To my surprise, the doctor defended her. I had thought he was going to thank me for bringing it to his attention. I could not imagine that the doctor would want a rude secretary on his staff. It turned out the person was his wife. Thankfully, he got a chuckle out of the whole thing.

Don't be too quick to judge. Some staff members are under a tremendous amount of stress at the front desk. They have a lot of multi-tasking to do. If you are kind to them, sometimes their attitude will turn around.

Seeing Multiple Doctors

Inform all of your doctors of all treatments and medications that you are getting elsewhere.

You may be in a situation where you have to get treatment from various doctors. In such a case, inform all your doctors of your medications and treatments. You don't want treatments to conflict. If you take simultaneous treatments, not only might they harm you, but you may not be able to sort out which treatment might be helping you. One doctor might encourage a specific treatment, while another may be opposed to it. One of my doctors said it was important that I drink orange juice fortified with calcium. A few days later, another doctor said I should not consume orange juice because of my yeast infections. What's good for one ailment is often bad for another.

Some treatments, such as cortisone injections, should be given only so many times within a certain timeframe. Keep your doctors informed about what treatments you are getting elsewhere.

Prior to any treatment, doctors should ask patients if they have had a similar treatment elsewhere and when. I have seen that question asked on forms that I filled out during my initial visits, but it's good to also discuss it during your visit.

Is Your Doctor Right?

Don't assume that your doctor is always correct.

A doctor once told me that I could get hand controls in my car the next day, if I wanted them. He said he drove his son's car that had them. I was surprised at his comment. In the state we both live in, a doctor must fill out a form about a patient's medical need for hand controls. That person then has to get trained and approved by the motor vehicle department. The facility that installs the hand controls has to know you passed the driving test. Your license has to indicate that you are legally approved to use hand controls. Hand controls cannot be placed in all vehicles; it depends upon a car's design and construction. Some people are licensed for driving with hand controls only around town (not highway), and some also have approval for highway driving. That doctor implied that I was not trying hard enough to get hand controls. I was merely trying to approach the installation of them legally.

I had the same set of dental x-rays read by four oral surgeons, and I was given four different interpretations of them.

One doctor might tell you there is no cure or treatment for your condition. Another facility or practitioner, however, may be able to help you.

Instincts

Follow your instincts. Encourage your doctors to understand the power of instincts.

It's important for doctors to recognize how valuable patients' instincts are. I regret not always following my instincts and listening to what a higher power was telling me. Not doing so got me into trouble. I let the fear and pressure from the disability reviewers get in the way of my gut feelings. The approach of the disability reviewers was not the best thing for me. I knew I could not work, but if I didn't follow through with the suggested surgeries, I could have lost my disability benefits. I took chances, hoping the surgeries would relieve my pain, despite my instincts, which told me otherwise.

Now, when I know a certain procedure is not good for me, I say no to it. There comes a point when your body simply cannot take any more surgical insults. You have to say yes to the health of your body.

It is my hope that more and more doctors will take patients' instincts seriously. Acceptance of instincts, and a respect for instincts, needs to be fully integrated into medical schools and training classes.

Does Your Doctor Put You to Work?

If your doctors are asking you to do something that you think their staff members should be doing, speak up.

Sometimes a doctor might ask you to investigate certain treatments or medicines. On occasion, I agree that it is a good way to proceed, but it would be best if the doctors had researchers on staff to do such work. It does not seem fair that a patient should be put to the task of finding things out that the doctor's office would be best doing. Other people told me they had been asked to track down labs, testing facilities, and clinical trials. The same thing happened to me on several occasions. I think it comes down to the offices not having the time or money to hire employees to do such research. If enough patients speak up about the problem, perhaps doctors will understand the need to assign such tasks to an appropriate staff member.

Can a Family Member Help?

Be honest with your practitioner about how much a family member can assist you.

Has your practitioner asked one of your family members to help with some of your home care? My husband was asked to do so on numerous occasions. If my husband took on what some practitioners wanted him to, it would have been another full-time job for him. I was seeing multiple practitioners, and all were giving my husband "homework" assignments. I had made each practitioner aware of the others, to avoid conflicts, and my husband's available time was limited. Let your practitioners know if they are unrealistic about what a significant other can handle. There may be times, however, that you do appreciate and want a significant other to help out. It depends on your situation.

In some situations, care handled by a licensed home-health aide is more appropriate than having a significant other help out. Other family members may have their own health problems that make it difficult for them to help you. If that's the case, inform your doctor of their conditions, so your doctor will understand your situation. Try to work out an arrangement that both you and your practitioner agree is best for your care.

Are House Calls Available?

If it's difficult for you to get out, ask your doctors if they know of doctors in your area who make house calls.

House calls are not the norm these days in the United States. Fortunately, the number of house calls is expected to grow, and a federal program known as "Independence at Home Act," encourages doctors to test the effectiveness of house calls.[16] The program allows Medicare beneficiaries suffering from multiple chronic conditions to receive primary care services in their homes, and the program is expected to reduce health-care costs.[17]

If you think about it, does it make sense that the person who is sick should always be the one having to travel to get help? I realize that sometimes patients must be seen at a facility where much of the medical equipment is. In certain instances, however, it makes more sense for a doctor to go to a patient's home. For example, one of my elderly relatives was once in a nursing home and needed a neurological exam. This person was bedridden, and she would have had to travel by ambulance to the doctor's office. She was told she might have to lie on a stretcher in the waiting room for more than an hour. It was finally decided that it was best for her not to go to the appointment because of the extreme measures it would take to get her there.

I am fully in favor of specialists and family doctors traveling to patients' homes for certain conditions and situations.

Many nursing homes have doctors that periodically stop in; however, they may not be the doctor to whom the patient was referred or the type of doctor the person needs to see.

Hooray to doctors who offer house calls!

Delays

Plan on everything taking longer than it should.

Over the years, I've found that most things I requested as a patient took much longer than I anticipated. Items I ordered from practitioners sometimes took weeks longer to arrive than I was told to expect. Pre-certification for insurance purposes occasionally took several weeks to fulfill rather than a few days. There are numerous situations where delays can happen. Don't assume that procedures are going to run smoothly.

The Experienced Patient

Use your experience to get yourself high-quality care.

The more you go to medical appointments, the more you will learn what you need to ask for, in order to receive the proper care you are entitled to. Your doctors may try to rush you or brush you off. Keep steadfast and stand up for what you are entitled to.

❧❧❧❧

After the Visit

Hanging Around after Your Appointment

If you depend upon transportation to pick you up, do your best to schedule appointments that do not extend into the office's lunchtime or closing time.

Many patients cannot drive and need to wait for a ride after their appointment. Most offices are very kind and allow you to sit in their waiting room until your ride shows up. Sometimes, however, you can tell that the receptionist is eager for your ride to appear. This is especially true if it's near lunchtime or closing time. It must be difficult for the office staff members if they are ready to close up and patients are still there. To avoid such situations, I sometimes schedule appointments in the early morning or early afternoon, to be assured that I am out of offices before closing times or lunch hours.

Parking Validations

Ask the office if it validates parking.

If you have to pay for parking, ask the receptionist at your doctor's office if he or she will validate your parking. By validating it, the office will pay the fee for you. One of my doctors always offered parking validation to his patients who were undergoing chemotherapy. When you park your car, if you get a slip for parking that does not say you must leave it in the car, take it to the office, which will need it to validate it. Most offices I visited did not validate, but some do, and it can't hurt to ask.

Can Your Doctor Dump You?

Don't assume that a physician has to accept or keep you as a patient.

In Connecticut, the state where I reside, doctors can tell you that they do not want to treat you anymore, because no laws say that they can or cannot do that.[18] Doctors in Connecticut who want to drop a patient do not have to give him or her advance notice, but the general practice is to give a thirty-day notice to allow for medication refills and for patients to find a new doctor.[19]

A doctor permanently dismissed my friend from his office because he didn't think he could appropriately treat her. Doctors may inform you that they think another doctor is more knowledgeable about your condition. A doctor might also feel that he or she does not have a good enough doctor-patient relationship with you to give the appropriate care.[20] Sometimes just having Medicare as a primary insurance plan can affect a doctor's decision to see you or not.

Contact the Department of Public Health in the state in which you reside, and ask if there are laws on these issues where you live.

Reporting Your Doctor

If your doctor acts unprofessionally, inform your insurance carrier.

One of my doctors made very unprofessional remarks to me during my visit with him. I'm not going to share the details of the event, but I called my insurance carrier as soon as I got home from the visit. Suffice it to say, the doctor's comments were truly shocking and outlandish. The doctor was on the insurance company's list of in-network and preferred doctors. The insurance company investigated my complaint and later removed the doctor from its list of network providers.

Inform your insurance carrier if you think you were treated in an extremely unprofessional manner. Your report will make the company aware of situations with providers that the company would otherwise not have known about. You can also inform the Department of Public Health in the state in which the doctor practices. Of course, if there was an extremely serious violation, or a situation posing a danger to yourself, you may also need to contact an attorney or the police.

Phone Calls to Your Doctor

Don't expect that your call will be returned immediately.

There may be times when you need to make a call to your doctors during office hours to ask a question. Most of my doctors returned my non-urgent calls around their lunchtime or in the early evening. It's best to make non-urgent calls later in the day, so you don't have to sit around all day waiting for a phone call. You get to know each doctor's style in returning calls. Some doctors squeeze in calls between their office visits.

Occasionally, I had to call my doctors on the weekend about issues that could not wait until Monday. Sometimes my calls from the early morning were not returned until late evening. If you truly have an emergency, call your local emergency number for help. If your need is not an emergency, but is rather urgent, inform the person who answers the doctor's phone.

On a rare occasion, a doctor may give you his or her cell number in case you need to call with questions that are not urgent. To my surprise, two of my doctors gave me their e-mail addresses to use for general questions and non-urgent matters. Don't abuse such a privilege. Use it only as instructed by your doctor.

When you call your doctors after hours, don't expect that they will necessarily be the one to call you back.

Another doctor might call you back instead of your own doctor. It all depends upon who is on call, especially when you call after normal business hours. That set-up can be frustrating; another doctor will not be as familiar with your medical history as your own doctor. That doctor might have a different conversational style from your regular doctor. On the positive side, it can give you an opportunity to get to know the other doctors. I've found some on-call doctors to be very kind and helpful.

Obtain Your Medical Records

Don't assume that the information in your medical records is correct. Request a copy of your medical records.

Your doctors take notes about what took place during your office visits. It's important that you review these notes for accuracy. Request a copy of your health records from your doctors and facilities that treated you. There may be a small fee for the records. Some offices waived the fee for me because I was on disability. If your doctors think that giving you the records will harm you in some way, they can withhold them. Usually the records have to be requested in writing, and sometimes there will be a form to fill out in order to obtain them. Ask your doctors what their procedures are to release their records to you.

I am astounded at the number of errors that I found in my doctors' notes over the last twenty-five years. One of my surgical reports noted that the doctor operated on my "breast" instead of my foot. I got a kick out of that. That particular error was most likely a simple clerical misunderstanding during translation from an audio recording of my doctor's notes. Notes stated that I had broken bones and diseases I did not have. Some stated the wrong limb as problematic. Rarely did my doctor's notes mention that I discussed adverse reactions to medications. Notes from phone conversations were especially brief. An entire paragraph in some notes about me stated the results of an examination it said I had. I was not, in fact, examined during the visit. I asked the doctor how he got the information, since I had not been examined. He admitted it was an error, and he speculated it was due to having used a template for the notes.

A template is only effective if the information entered into it is accurate. Computerized templates sometimes assume that work performed during a prior office visit was repeated at the subsequent visit.[21] When a patient's name is entered, the computer sometimes duplicates information from the prior visit, and uses the current date.[22]

It is also important to get notes from a hospital where you had surgery. If you have an implant or any device in you, find out the manufacturer and the specific name of the product. Ask if the surgeon purposely left metal staples or clips in you. This information is critical if you later have to get a test done or if there is a recall of your medical device. If you wait too many years to get the notes, you run the risk of a facility having discarded them.

I first became aware of the importance of accurate notes when I was at my chiropractor's office. I overheard several patients talking about the errors they found in their practitioners' notes. Some thought they had been denied disability benefits due to the errors. I can relate to what they said because the notes about me also lacked the detail that disability reviewers needed.

When I've told my doctors that their notes need to be specific and legible for disability purposes, they sometimes thought I was overly concerned. I think physicians should be trained on how to write notes for disability statuses.

Inaccurate notes are one of the most unfair things that can happen to a patient. If the notes reflect a disease you do not have, or identify the wrong limb, they can affect you when applying for life or disability insurance. The notes have a huge impact on your disability status. Incorrect notes can also lead to a potentially dangerous situation if another doctor acts upon false information in the notes. Patients need to be on top of this, and insist on accuracy.

Some patients may not want to receive their notes. Perhaps they are afraid of what they will find out. They might also be concerned that they won't understand the terminology. Still others may not want to take the time to obtain the notes. Patients might also feel that requesting the notes reflects a distrust of their doctors, especially if they've seen their practitioner for many years. Patients must decide for themselves whether obtaining notes is in their best interest or not.

Some physicians did not like that I obtained the notes, but I knew I was smart to get them and check them. Some doctors and hospitals don't think that it's in patients' best interest to receive notes, so these facilities will levy hefty charges to copy the notes.[23] Some doctors require that patients read the notes in front of them.[24] Perhaps physicians dislike the extra paperwork involved in copying patient notes, or worry that discussing the notes will take up precious time during office visits.

The *OpenNotes* project, launched in the summer of 2010, evaluated the impact of obtaining physicians' notes.[25] My understanding is that this was a twelve-month study in which more than one hundred primary care physicians and about 25,000 patients volunteered to participate.[26] It will be interesting to learn how practitioners, patients, and medical facilities react to the results of the study.

When I discover incorrect notes, I write a letter to my doctor with the corrected changes and ask that it be kept in my file. Review your patient rights on having changes made to the notes at www.hhs.gov/.[27]

Physicians are encouraged to use electronic medical records. The Obama administration declared that penalties could begin in 2015 for providers that haven't adopted the use of electronic medical records.[28] Although electronic records can be beneficial, we must be concerned with the accuracy, security, and privacy of those records.

Medical Records for Sale

Write to legislatures if you have concerns about the sale of medical records.

Did you know that your medical records may have been up for sale? Your records are helpful to researchers who have broad access to them despite privacy laws.[29] Congress passed the Health Information Technology for Economic and Clinical Health Act to reinforce the security of records.[30]

Privacy laws are complex and are updated at various times to prevent loopholes for marketers and researchers to latch on to. Consult an attorney if you want more information about the sale of medical records. Privacy laws are too complex for laypersons to keep current with or interpret.

We must ensure that the security of our medical records keeps pace with the electronic processing of them. If you have concerns with the sale of medical records, write to your state legislature and Congress.

Supplies and Supplements

Don't assume that you have to buy your supplies and supplements at your doctor's office.

Your doctors might suggest that you purchase an item or supplement they sell. You might be able to buy the item cheaper elsewhere, but be sure you are getting the exact product your doctor wants you to have. Your doctor might have a reason for wanting you to use a product made by a specific manufacturer. Also ask your doctor how necessary it is for you to have an item before you spend the money on it. I think some practitioners felt as if they were at least trying to have me leave their office with something tangible. Later on, many practitioners did not even remember that they suggested certain things to me.

Be sure the supplements that you receive have been properly stored. Inform your doctor of all supplements that you are taking.

Some supplements need refrigeration, even prior to opening them. If so, be sure the facility where you buy those supplements has not left them sitting out on an unrefrigerated shelf. I ask facilities if certain supplements have been refrigerated properly. Bring a cooler to your appointment to put refrigerated medical supplements in for the ride home.

Make your doctor aware of all supplements you are taking. Talk to your doctor and pharmacist to be sure that your supplements are not conflicting with other medicines you are taking. Doctors and pharmacists may not have all the answers to your supplement questions, because so many supplements are available these days. More research should be done to prove the effectiveness and side effects of supplements.

Ask your practitioners if they have the necessary supplies on hand for treatments they suggest you have done in the near future.

You might assume that your doctor's office has necessary supplies on hand. One of my dentists did not have a case for the retainer he had made me. He and his facility provide excellent service overall, so I was surprised. It shows how easy it is, even for a place who gives great service, to run out of supplies. I had to walk out of his office holding the retainer in my hand.

One of my doctors had to catheterize me in her office prior to each of my chemotherapy sessions. The chemotherapy was to be given a few hours later at another facility. When I arrived at my doctor's office to be catheterized, the nurse said she did not have the type of catheter she needed for me. The doctor had to send someone out to buy one while I waited on the examining table. That doctor also had provided me with great service over the years. Things get so hectic at facilities that staffers can lose track of what needs to be restocked. Offices and hospitals need to take inventory more frequently. Perhaps the office ordered the items, but they got delayed during shipping. It's possible that the delays originated with the manufacturers. No matter what, not having the proper supplies on hand can have a negative impact on a patient's treatment.

If you have an important treatment coming up, consider asking your doctor or nurse if they have all the supplies on hand. I think that some practitioners found my asking intrusive, but others appreciated it and were glad I reminded them.

Medical Letters from Your Doctors

If your doctor is writing a medical letter for you for insurance purposes, check with the insurance company to see what key points it needs in the letter. Review your doctor's letter.

There may be times that you'll need a letter of medical necessity from your doctor for insurance purposes; for example, suppose your doctor suggests that you get a leg brace. Call your medical insurance carrier to find out if it needs a letter from your doctor that states why the equipment is medically necessary for you. If the insurance company needs a letter, ask if there are key points your doctor should address in the letter. Relay that information to your doctor. You must be honest. If the key points that your insurance carrier wants addressed are not included in the letter, you run the risk of being denied approval for the equipment or having the process take longer. The insurance company may then need more information from your doctor.

Review your doctor's letter, if possible, before it's sent out. I have found numerous grammatical errors and missing information in doctors' letters. Some of the grammatical errors made a critical difference as to how certain sentences could be interpreted. When I found errors, I asked my doctors to fix them, which put me in a precarious situation, because I had to put pressure on my doctors to get the corrected letter back to me quickly. Otherwise, I could miss the deadline date by which the insurance company needed to receive the letter. Getting a good letter on time from your practitioners is one of the most challenging tasks a patient has to coordinate. Be very persistent to get these letters from your doctors.

If you have special needs that require attention, ask your doctor to write a letter to your other practitioners and request that it be kept in their files.

If you have a medical condition that makes it difficult for you to sit through certain medical or dental procedures, ask your doctor to write a letter explaining your limitations. Then, you can ask your other practitioners to keep that letter in your file. My doctor wrote a letter about my bladder problem so that my other doctors would understand why I need to get up often during procedures. It was very helpful and gave me more credibility when I told my other practitioners about my bladder condition.

Experimental Treatments

Use caution when undergoing experimental treatments.

Sometimes your doctor may offer a treatment that is considered experimental. I avoid them, because usually insurance companies will not pay for experimental procedures. If you decide to pay on your own, use caution. If you later have a medical condition that is thought to have been brought on by that experimental treatment, most likely your insurance will not cover that either.

Several years ago, I found out that I had been part of a medical experiment, and I didn't even know it. After my ovarian cancer surgery, the nurse at the hospital put special cuffs on my legs to prevent blood clots. Some of the patients got these particular cuffs, and some patients received another type of cuff. I really liked the cuffs, but I had no idea that I was part of an experiment. I discovered that several weeks later, when I called the hospital to find out what the brand name of the cuffs was. I felt that they had helped some of the problems I had with my legs, and I was considering buying a pair. I don't know the legality of experiments like that. Suppose it was an experiment I wanted no part of? Perhaps I had unknowingly signed paperwork allowing it. This is another reason why patients should be given ample time to review forms pertaining to their surgery.

When Your Practitioners Can't Connect

You might need to remind your practitioners that they were going to call another practitioner about your care.

There may be times when your practitioners say that they will call another one of your practitioners regarding a certain aspect of your care. This has happened to me on several occasions, and I was often told they were unable to connect. It can be difficult for some practitioners to reach each other when they are seeing patients all day. If your case is an emergency, most likely there will be a system in place to allow interruptions for such phone calls. It's frustrating when practitioners can't connect within a reasonable time, and it can hold up a patient's treatment. It doesn't hurt to ask your practitioner if they were able to reach another practitioner they told you they were going to talk to. They can get so busy that they forget they were going to place the call. Some practitioners were actually glad that I reminded them.

Have an Emergency Plan

Develop a plan for natural disasters.

If you take medication or have a chronic health condition, it's important to have supplies on hand in case an emergency arises. For example, suppose you have to leave your home due to a storm or other crisis. Pack a suitcase with clothing, flashlights, personal supplies, medications that you need, and other supplies ahead of time. Also think about where you will go and how you will get there. If you can't drive, what mode of transportation will you use to get to your destination?

If you use a wheelchair, be sure the place you are going to has wheelchair access.

Be sure you have a means to recharge your cell phone, if you have one. It may be your only lifeline if your land phone goes out.

Talk to neighbors, relatives, friends, and others you depend upon about your plan. Gather their phone numbers and keep them with you. Also obtain the phone numbers of your local shelter, electric company, police, and fire department.

If family members live alone, have someone check on them periodically.

It's a good idea to have a relative or neighbor check-in on an elderly person or person with a chronic health condition. Perhaps you can agree to call the person once a day at a certain time. If there is no answer, you will be alerted that something may be wrong.

Some people wear a necklace or bracelet that has an emergency alert button on it. When they press it, a facility will immediately be notified that there is a problem. Other people use a speaker system that allows them to yell out and be heard at a designated facility. You have to be within a certain distance of the speaker to be heard, though.

Some facilities will call a neighbor, officially selected in advance to be a contact, to check on you if you press a button or call for help. Otherwise, they will send the proper emergency personnel to help you.

Some families install a webcam or other computer device for visual monitoring of their loved ones.

❦❦❦❦

Prescriptions and Tests

Prescriptions

Examine the label on your medication's container to be sure you received the proper medication and dose that your doctor prescribed.

Haven't we all received prescription slips from our doctors that are not legible? I rarely receive one in which a doctor filled in my date of birth or address. I think all that information should be completed by the doctor. Otherwise, patients could give their prescription to someone else with the same name. That's probably a rare event, but I can imagine pain pill prescriptions may be especially prone to such abuse. I think doctors should make a practice of calling prescriptions in to drugstores. Some pharmacies have an electronic method that allows submission of typed prescriptions, which can cut down on errors from poor handwriting.[31]

When you pick up a prescription, thoroughly check the label on the bottle to be sure you were given the correct medication and dosage. I even count the number of pills to be sure the pharmacy put the correct number in the bottle. If I can't read my doctor's handwriting on a prescription, I'll ask my doctor to clarify what he or she wrote. That way, I can be sure my pharmacist interpreted my doctor's handwriting correctly. Some pharmacies require that you pick up your prescription within a certain number of days. Otherwise, they will put the medication back into their stock.

When you are picking up a new medication, ask the pharmacist if you should avoid exposure to sunlight while you are on the medication. Some medications cause skin reactions and other problems if you are in the sun. Also, ask if there are certain foods you should not take with your prescription. Inform your pharmacist of any supplements you are taking.

Your pharmacy might not always have your medication in stock when you need it. If you urgently need a medication that is not available at your pharmacy, ask the pharmacist to recommend another shop that may have it on hand immediately. If you cannot obtain it soon enough, tell your doctor.

As I mentioned before, if you are seeing multiple doctors, inform them of prescriptions that other doctors have given you. It's critical that they be aware of all prescriptions you are getting elsewhere. You don't want medications to overlap or interact in a negative way.

Shop around for the best prices. Consider getting your medications via mail order.

Pharmacies vary in their prices for medications. I use a drugstore that honors my American Automobile Association (AAA) membership. This costs quite a bit less than at another pharmacy down the street, which does not honor AAA. Also ask your pharmacist if the store offers other discount programs for generic drugs. It's worthwhile to shop around for the best prices.

Some retail stores offer discount programs for prescriptions. Find out if the store charges a fee for such services.

Your medical insurance carrier may offer to mail your medications directly to your home. This is convenient, and it sometimes costs less than at a local drugstore.

Some people are hesitant to use mail order because they are afraid their medication will get lost in the mail or arrive late. If your medication did not arrive in a timely manner, ask your doctor to prescribe a small quantity until you finally get your order. Some doctors will do that for you. Insurance, however, may not cover such a small quantity. My medications have never been lost in the mail, and I have always gotten them on time.

It's important to ask the manufacturer what temperatures the medicine can tolerate. You don't want it to be subjected to improper temperatures during transit time or while it's in your mailbox. I called regarding a medicine that was delivered to me when it was extremely hot outside. The manufacturer's representative told me that it should not be subjected to temperatures over approximately 77 degrees Fahrenheit.[32] She also gave me a phone number to another corporate department that my pharmacist could call to get more detailed information. My pharmacist called and found out that the medication can tolerate a temperature range of 86-114 degrees Fahrenheit for up to six months.[33] I'm glad I checked, or I may have tossed out the prescription based on the first person's response.

If you use a hot tub, be sure that any transdermal patches you wear can withstand the temperature of the water. I've also been told it's not good to store medications in the bathroom. Ask your pharmacist or manufacturer what the ideal temperature and conditions are for your medication.

Find out if you are eligible to get your prescription for free.

If you don't have prescription coverage, or are under great financial stress, ask your doctors if they can suggest reputable places from which you can possibly get your prescriptions for free. Ask manufacturers if they offer free prescriptions programs that you can apply for. Sometimes you can find coupons online for medications that are considered cosmetic. Cosmetic medications are usually not covered by insurance. Doctors are sometimes very generous in giving out samples. You can also call hospitals for help in getting free medications.

Take care not to mistake one medication for another. Properly dispose of expired medications.

Check your medications periodically to be sure they haven't expired. If you have to throw them out, call your town's hazardous waste department to ask how you should properly discard them. I've noticed that the prescription labels from my pharmacy always note that my prescriptions expire within one year from the date I filled them. Some prescriptions for creams and gels have an expiration date on their tubes, however, that is much later. If you have any questions about when your prescription expires, ask your pharmacist. A pharmacist told me that pills should never be used beyond the date of the pharmacy label, but creams might be effective until the expiration date on the tube.[34]

Develop a system that allows you to clearly identify your medications. Most pharmacies sell containers that make it convenient to organize your pills, helping to avoid mix-ups. It's easy to mistakenly take the wrong pill. I transferred one of my prescriptions to another pharmacy and still had some of the old medication in my closet. When I picked up the new medication, I realized it had different packaging. Apparently, that drugstore uses a different manufacturer for the same medication. I kept forgetting they were the same medication because the box that they came in looked so different. That made me realize how easy it is to confuse medications, especially when you are in a hurry.

You also have to be concerned about counterfeit medications. Counterfeit medications are fraudulent and may not have the correct ingredients even though the packaging and labeling looks genuine. It's not easy to spot them. You might suspect a counterfeit if your medication is not working for you the way it normally does. If you have suspicions that you have a counterfeit medicine, tell your pharmacist who may have ways to spot differences between a real and counterfeit medicine.

Prescription mix-ups happen in hospitals, too. A friend of mine was almost given a medicine meant for the patient next to her. Fortunately, she discovered the error in time.

Keep a list of your allergies, as well as the medications that you take. Hang the list in a visible place at home.

It's a good idea to write down your allergies and any medications you take. Write down the doses of the medications and times you take the medications. Hang the list in a visible place in your home so others may see it, in case you have an emergency medical situation. Do that for all of your family members. I also keep a copy of my medical history in my purse and my car.

There are online resources to help you keep track of your medications. If you use such resources, be sure you also have a printed copy of your medication list hanging in a visible place.

Reporting a Reaction to a Medication

Don't let physicians dismiss your reactions to medications.

I once called the manufacturer of a medicine that I reacted to. The representative, who answered the phone, asked for my name and address and then transferred me to another facility. The person to whom I was transferred wanted paperwork from my doctors verifying that the medication caused the reaction, or that there was a strong possibility that it did.

The problem was that my doctors dismissed my reaction to the medication. So, after I went through all the bureaucracy, I was at a dead end because my physicians would not substantiate my reaction to the medication. That attitude from doctors puts patients in a dilemma. On the one hand, I understand that the agency that tracks reactions needs to have information from doctors. It gives patients' concerns credibility. On the other hand, patients have little recourse.

I also called a manufacturer to get a list of ingredients in its adhesive electrodes to which my skin reacted badly. The company representative told me the ingredients, and she said it was necessary that the company file my call as a complaint. The representative sent me a pre-paid mailer so that I could mail her a sample electrode. She then sent the electrode to another area of the company to be sure that particular lot of electrodes did not have defects. The company contacted me once their investigation was complete.

If you want to find out the ingredients of something you reacted to, keep in mind that it can turn into a lengthy process. Perhaps that's why some doctors dismiss patients' reactions to medications. Acknowledging reactions to medications would result in lots of paperwork for doctors. Doctors might also think that they cannot prove that a certain medication caused a reaction and that other variables make it difficult to pinpoint a reaction to one specific medication.

Doses of Medicine

If you are reluctant to take a certain medication because of potential side effects, ask your doctor if you can start with a lower dose. Never take a lower dose without asking your doctor.

If my doctor wants me to start a new medication, I ask if I can begin with the lowest dose to see how I react to it. It's critical that you follow your doctor's advice regarding dosing requirements. Certain doses may be necessary to prevent complications, some of which could be life-threatening.

I always ask my pharmacist and my doctor if my pills can be split in half. Some pills should not be split, as that could cause serious problems. Never split a pill unless your doctor says it's okay. Don't open or split a capsule or extended release medication.

Your doctor needs to know if the dose you took was other than what he or she prescribed. You need to be honest with your doctor as to whether you followed the directions regarding a medication.

If you react to a particular medicine, inform your doctor. If your reaction is life-threatening, call your local emergency number for help. I took a pill given to me for neurological reasons. Per my doctor's approval, I took only one-fourth of the dose. An hour later, I experienced strange flashing of lights in my eyes after looking at the sun. I went to my eye doctor who agreed it was possible that I would be left with such symptoms due to the medicine.

Sometimes there are side effects that you will eventually get used to, so stopping the medication abruptly is not necessarily the right thing to do.

Ask your doctor if you need periodic blood tests.

Some medications can affect the liver or other organs of the body. Medications can affect the nutrients in your body, as well. When your doctor first gives you a prescription for medication, ask him or her if a periodic blood test is necessary. If it is required, ask how often you should have it done. Even the best of doctors can forget important tests.

Consider a compounding pharmacy for certain medications and for unusual doses of medications.

If a regular pharmacy can't get you the dose you want, consider a compounding pharmacy, although this might be expensive. Compounding pharmacies can make up a unique dose of medicine for you, provided you have a prescription from your doctor. I've found compounding pharmacists to be very helpful and willing to take the time to answer questions.

Medicine with No Side Effects

Don't rely on a doctor to tell you the side effects of a medication.

A doctor once handed me a prescription and told me it had absolutely no side effects. I exclaimed that it must have some. He replied, "No, zero." I knew it was not true. How could it possibly have no side effects, unless it was a placebo? I asked my pharmacist for the manufacturer's sheet that lists the side effects. It showed a long list of side effects. I think that doctors rely too much on what salespeople tell them or that doctors don't have time to research the side effects of medications. Many of my doctors suggested I talk to a pharmacist regarding my medication questions, because my doctors thought the pharmacist was more knowledgeable in that regard. Even if side effects are rare, I want to know what they are, and I want to be the one to determine what risks I am willing to take.

During chemotherapy, an anti-nausea medicine actually made me feel nauseated. I looked up the side effects and one of them was nausea. Sometimes the side effects are the same as, or worse than, the original discomfort. I realize some patients are significantly helped by anti-nausea medication. I just find it humorous that an anti-nausea drug can cause nausea.

Why Aren't You Taking More Medications?

Don't be surprised if your doctors wonder why you are not taking more medications.

Years ago, nurses and doctors seemed surprised when I told them that the only medication I take is estrogen. I knew this partially had to do with the disability factor; they were most likely thinking that I didn't want to try and get better. I previously tried all medicines prescribed to me. Most of them had side effects that led me to discontinue them. I am more cautious now about taking medications. I am not saying to stop your medication(s) or not to take any. Your doctor should examine the need for each medication and find out if there are less-invasive ways to approach your treatment.

I think genetics plays a role in how we react to medicine and that much of our reaction depends upon our size and weight. I'm very petite, so I sometimes ask my doctors for a small dose. I usually do fine on just a quarter of the dose of pain medications. Doctors should take size into account and keep track of poor reactions. If your doctor prescribes pain medicine for you, consider asking if you can take just enough of it to take the edge off, but not so much that you will become drowsy. There are some medications for which it is critical you take the full amount.

There might be times that your dentist suggests you take an anti-inflammatory after a dental procedure. After one root canal, a hygienist told me to take two anti-inflammatories when I got home. I thought she meant for pain, so I told her I would rather not take the pills. My dentist happened to be walking by just at that moment and overheard me. He came into the room and said that he wanted me to take the pills to keep the inflammation down. Sometimes, taking the medicine is the best thing to do.

Privacy

Be aware of how your personal information is used.

I recently read that some insurance companies use a FICO Medication Adherence Score to determine how likely a person is to take their medicine.[35] The scores will help identify patients who could benefit from follow-up phone calls or e-mails regarding their medicine.[36] The FICO medication score uses public data, not medical history, to make its predictions. I find the use of this score intrusive.

Free Samples

Always check the expiration date of sample medications.

If your doctor gives you free samples, check their expiration date. Some of my practitioners gave me expired samples. I was always amazed when my practitioners did not look at expiration dates before they gave samples to me. Ask your doctors if the samples are the same dose that they would have given you had you been given a prescription for it. You also have to remember your doctor's instructions for taking the medicine before you use samples. They won't have the directions on them like the ones you pick up at your pharmacy.

Test Results

Ask your doctor to call you even if your test results are negative.

I think patients should be notified whether their test results are positive or negative. What if the office forgot to call you when the test result was positive? Ask your doctor's office to call you even if your test results are negative. A friend of mine was told she'd only get a call if the results where positive. Many weeks went by before the office realized it had forgotten to inform her that the results were positive. This caused significant problems for her that could have been avoided. Some offices mail a card showing the results, or they send you an e-mail.

I used to confuse the meaning of the terms positive and negative regarding test results. I thought positive meant that the results were fine. That's because I think of the word positive in a favorable context. It's the opposite, though, unless you want to get pregnant and your test is positive! A positive test result means they found something out of the normal range for which they may have a concern. A negative test result means the results were within a normal range.

Your doctor might spot positive results, but in the context and interpretation of the entire test, may rightfully assure you that there is nothing to be concerned about. So don't panic if you see something showing as positive. Doctors should explain what positive and negative results mean, especially to a young patient who has never been to a doctor before. Such information can be helpful to a teenager getting her first gynecological exam and Pap smear, for example.

If you have an appointment with your doctor to discuss your test results, call the office a few days before your appointment to be sure they have received the results. I've arrived at appointments, only to find that my doctors did not have the test results. Some receptionists told me they had the results, but when I got to my appointment, the information was not there.

Don't ignore borderline test results.

A pet peeve of mine is when doctors quickly scan test results just looking in the "positive" column. One of my doctors told me that he just looks in the positive column. A test could show a negative result that is only one number away from being positive. I had a blood test for which a number higher than 99 would have meant an abnormal result for the specific item my doctor tested me for. My number was exactly 99, which meant it was very close to being positive. My doctor was very good about taking this borderline number into account. She told me to get tested again, in the near future. I respected her attention to detail.

The number ranges for determining a positive or negative result may vary from lab to lab. My friend saved a copy of her blood test results for a specific test. Over time, she noticed that the numbers were creeping up to an almost positive result. She brought this to the attention of her doctors. It turned out she had a blood disorder that may not have been diagnosed without her attentiveness and proactive approach.

Blood Tests and Labs

If you think too much blood is being drawn for tests, talk to your doctor about it. Some labs take more blood than others for the same test.

After getting several bloods tests over the years, I noticed that some labs took more blood than others for the same test. I went in person to three labs with the same lab slip. I asked the technicians approximately how many tubes of blood they would take. I was amazed at the differences in their answers, despite the fact that all labs showed me the same size tube. One lab told me they would take two tubes of blood, another said three to four, and one even said five. I asked them why the number of tubes taken varies so much from lab to lab. The responses were mixed. Some said that's just how they do it, and others said they take extra blood in case it spills. Tube sizes can vary at labs, so a better question to ask is how many cubic centimeters will be taken. A cubic centimeter is a measurement of volume. Discuss any concerns or questions you have about this with your doctor.

The amount of blood is important to me because I had an attack of shingles brought on by too much blood being drawn. When I expressed my concerns about the amount of blood being drawn, the technician laughed at me. My instincts told me that too much blood was being taken. I came home from the test unusually tired. Soon after, I broke out with shingles. My doctor said that taking so much blood had probably lowered my immune system and caused the shingles outbreak. When I told my other doctors about it, they dismissed it.

I now choose labs that take less blood, and I tell them not to take more than is absolutely necessary. I usually check with the lab a few days before drawing the blood to see approximately how much will be drawn. I definitely check with the lab if several items are checked on a lab slip. If you have concerns about such issues, talk to your doctor prior to undergoing a blood test.

Prior to surgical procedures patients are usually required to have blood drawn during pre-admission testing. When prescribing pre-admission testing, I think doctors should take into account if patients had blood taken within the last few months. You don't want too much blood to be taken within a certain timeframe; this could lower your immune system and impede your recovery from surgery.

When doctors prescribe blood tests, I think they should ask patients if their other doctors also recently ordered blood tests for them. This not only prevents duplicate testing, but it also ensures that not too much blood is being drawn within a certain timeframe. Keep your doctor informed of other tests you recently had, or will be having.

Labs should verify that you followed the exact instructions for the test. It is critical you do as told to get an accurate test reading. If you have concerns about fasting, discuss them with your doctor prior to the day of the test. Ask your doctor if you should stop your medications or supplements prior to your blood test.

My doctors and the labs sometimes disagreed regarding fasting requirements. Sometimes, doctors told me I didn't have to fast, but the lab technician said I did. If a conflict exists, tell your doctor what the lab said. Your doctor may have a reason for his or her instructions. Be sure you clearly understand whether you should fast from liquids, solid foods, or both liquids and solid foods. Be sure you know the number of hours that you should fast.

On a few occasions, labs have lost my test results. It's so frustrating to have to repeat the test.

Be patient with lab workers.

Years ago, labs usually had a person at the front desk who input insurance information and another who drew blood. Recently, I've noticed that one person often performs both types of tasks. This puts excessive time demands on lab workers, and it also results in a longer waiting time for patients. If a patient's lab slip has numerous items on it, it will take the lab worker a long time to input the information into the computer. If the lab slip is not legible, the worker will also have to make calls to verify information.

I think it's unfair and unreasonable that labs expect one worker to do the task of two or more people.

Don't assume you must go to the lab your doctor uses.

Some doctors gave me lab slips with the name of a particular lab on them, without asking me what lab I use. My insurance carrier, however, sometimes pays a higher benefit for services at a lab other than the ones my doctors suggest. Discuss such issues with your doctors.

Some of my doctors insisted I use the lab they recommended, because they trust the services at that lab, and they were used to interpreting that lab's results. Other doctors didn't care what lab I went to, and they agreed to give me another slip with the correct lab name on it.

Some doctors didn't change the name of the lab on the slips, despite agreeing that I could use a different lab. Some labs would not accept my lab slip without their name on it; others didn't care what name was listed on my slip.

Don't ignore your practitioners' advice regarding labs. Some labs may be more highly skilled than others in performing certain tests.

Retail Clinics

Find out about the retail clinics in your area.

Medical clinics are found at many drugstores and retailers. They are becoming more common for acute conditions such as ear-aches, poison ivy, and sprains, although some will not treat infants under a certain age.[37] I can image that customers like the convenience of retail clinics. Some health insurers have added clinics in malls.[38] I prefer to see my own family physician. It's not a bad idea, though, to check out the clinics in your area. You might find that they come in handy if you can't get an appointment soon enough with your doctor.

Keep in mind that retail clinics are not a substitute for the overall care you receive at your doctor's office, and they are not a substitute for the emergency room. You can work out a plan with your doctor as to how you can best utilize such services if the need arises.

Urine Tests

Clearly label your urine sample to avoid mix-ups.

Many of us have had to leave a urine sample during a visit with our doctor. Some offices didn't ask me to write my initials or name on the sample, even when there was another sample in the same room as mine. I put my name on it anyway. I think there should be an identifying label for each patient. The nurse could, for instance, pull a pre-labeled sticker from your file and place it on the cup before you give the sample. It would include the patient's full name and date of birth. It could lessen the chance of a mix-up. I legibly write my full name and date of birth on my samples, even if I'm told to just put my first name or initials on them. What if another person with the same first name happened to leave their sample too? Play it safe, and include the detail.

If you have to drop a sample off at a lab, be sure you know of any requirements for refrigeration. Some samples will not be good if left at room temperature for too long. If you do the test at home, be sure you follow all instructions and know how quickly you must get your sample to the lab. If it requires refrigeration, make the lab technician aware of that when you drop it off. I usually call the lab, before I drop off my sample, and ask them exactly where I should leave my sample if no one is at the desk. I also do that to be sure they know to look for it, so it's not sitting out too long.

Magnetic Resonance Imaging (MRI)

MRI facilities tell you what you can and cannot wear or bring into the testing area. Follow those directions fully.

Upon arrival to some of my MRI tests, the technicians did not ask if I had taken off my jewelry. This surprised me, as they should be sure you are not wearing any metal. Anyone going in the room with you must follow the facility's rules in terms of what they can and cannot have on them.

One doctor said that my mother should not get a MRI test due to the metal plate in her hip, but another doctor mistakenly scheduled her for one. Apparently, he had not looked at her history in detail.

Bring the appropriate clothing for the test. The facility where you are having the MRI will usually call you before the test date and go over such details with you. Sometimes the facility will furnish you with a gown to wear. I think all patients should be required to put the facility's gown on, instead of wearing their own clothes. If not, I think all clothing should be thoroughly checked by the MRI technician. Otherwise, a person could have accidentally left something metal on them and not realized it. Due to the high magnetic forces, such items can cause serious injury. Most of my MRI technicians only asked me if I had any metal on me. One place, however, was excellent and had me stand under a device that detects metal. Prior to your MRI, inform the technician of any metal or artificial apparatuses, rings, implants, contacts lenses, snaps, earrings, makeup, tattoos, nail polish, etc., that you may have on or in you. The facilities I went to had me complete a questionnaire regarding that.

My husband was allowed to wear his contact lenses during a MRI, but only because they were not tinted. Never wear your contact lenses during a MRI unless the technician says you can.

Some places have special headphones that you can wear to drown out the noises from the MRI machine. The facility might, instead, offer you earplugs to wear. Do not bring your own head-phones or earplugs. Use only what the facility gives you or allows you to use.

Once, while I was getting a MRI, the technician assured me that he would hear me if I shouted out to him for help. Towards the last ten minutes of the test, I yelled out to him because my bladder pressure was so severe that I felt nauseous. He didn't hear me. Ask the technician to check the sound system. Some places will offer you a buzzer to press if you need help. If you can't tolerate being enclosed in a MRI machine due to claustrophobia or other reasons, ask your doctor if you can get an open MRI.

Ask your doctor if there is a specific radiologist that should interpret your MRI.

Another factor to consider is which radiologist will analyze your MRI. Some are more skilled than others in looking for certain dis-orders. Some of my doctors thought a certain test was worthwhile only if a certain radiologist interpreted it.

Ask for a copy of your MRI.

Many places will give you a copy of your MRI after your test is done. Some places gave me a copy without my doctor autho-rizing it. Other places required my doctor's authorization for me to get a copy. Ask the facility ahead of time what their requirements are if you want one. Keep the copy in your file at home in case a need for it arises in the future.

I like having a copy of the MRI because sometimes I want to get a second opinion from another doctor. For example, after a MRI of my foot, I found out about a doctor in New York who is highly skilled at reading MRI results for the condition I have. I paid him a few hundred dollars to read the results of my MRI because his opinion was worth it to me.

If you are picking up your original radiological films from a facility, don't leave them lying around in your car for hours in the hot sun or freezing temperatures. Take care not to get fingerprints or scratches on them. The place you picked them up from will want them back. They actually own the original films. These days, many facilities send CDs of MRIs to doctors to view on their computer. They are certainly less clumsy than films, and they have less risk of being damaged or smudged.

Find out what type of MRI machine is best for your condition.

Some facilities offer stronger MRI machines that can detect a lot of detail. They can sometimes reveal more than the common 1.5 Tesla strength machines. That is another example of why doctors should not be quick to judge patients as having a psychiatric disorder just because nothing shows up on the test. It's possible the MRI machine with the higher magnetic strength will reveal something that a lower magnetic strength could not. For some conditions, a radiologist told me, a stronger MRI machine may not necessarily find more. The strength that was suggested for my condition was a 3 Tesla (3T) MRI machine. For some ailments, the 3T might not make much of a difference. Certain medical reasons might prevent the use of a stronger MRI for some people. Your doctor may have a very good reason for sending you to a particular place and using a certain machine.

Some of my doctors were very good about examining the MRI strength options available to me. If your doctor does not take that initiative, consider calling facilities and asking them what MRI machines they have. Then, share that information with your doctor to determine which place is the best for you to have the testing done. I had a problem getting a MRI of my foot at one facility because their machine was quite narrow. My feet required an unusual set-up, which resulted in the need for a wider MRI. I was able to find a facility with a wider machine, which made it possible for me to have the test. You also have to take into account what facilities your insurance will pay for. Some tests tend to be more expensive at hospitals than at outpatient facilities. Perhaps this is because hospitals have such high overhead costs.

Some MRI centers offer testing facilities in various locations. Not all locations necessarily do MRI testing with contrast injections. Sometimes doctors will order a test with a contrast injection. Be sure the facility you are going to is equipped to handle your needs. Usually the doctor's office takes care of all that. Because of the number of clerical errors I've encountered over the years, I always call on my own to double-check. I even ask the MRI center if they have skilled people to put the needle in my arm for the injection. They often have trouble getting it to stay in my veins. I like to know that a very skilled person is going to do my test.

Some places told me that all of their technicians are equipped to handle difficult veins. I've not found that to be true. I ran into trouble during a stress test years ago. After several attempts, a technician could not get the needle to stay in my vein. She told me she was not very experienced. I had to wait a long time before the hospital tracked down someone who was skilled enough to get the needle in my vein.

A Technician's Attitude

If you are happy with a technician's service, let the facility know. If you thought a technician was rude, inform a supervisor.

Most technicians that I had were very kind when preparing or giving me a test. Sometimes I had trouble getting my body to go into the exact position they wanted. Most technicians were very patient and tried to find alternative approaches to positioning me. It made everything go smoothly. On occasion, I've had technicians who were not patient. A little patience and empathy from a technician can go a long way in making the procedure go better for everyone. It can help to put patients at ease and alleviate their fears.

A Technician's Experience

Speak up if you think a technician is being careless.

Have you ever been in the middle of a test and wondered if the technician knew what he or she was doing? I experienced that on just one occasion. The test was supposed to take approximately ten minutes. It was a test I had several times before without any problem. This particular technician was not trained in the software, and she kept making calls to understand how to use it. Nearly an hour later, she was ready to give me the test, but was not certain how to adjust the machine to have it scan over me. I sat up on the table and politely told her that I was not going to continue with the test. If something does not seem right, don't be afraid to speak up.

Is the Test Necessary?

Ask your doctor how critical a test is and whether the results will truly help determine your care.

Over the years, I discovered that my doctors sometimes used insurance guidelines to determine how often I should get a specific test done. One doctor told me it was imperative that I get a certain test done annually. When I came in the following year for the test, he seemed surprised. He said the test is now only needed every two years because that is how often my insurance company will pay for it. It's funny how the urgency of a test can change so quickly based on what an insurance plan will cover. A medical practitioner once told me that when a facility gets a new machine, they sometimes increase the testing frequency to help pay for the machine. I can't speak to the validity of his comment, but it makes sense to me that a facility may do that.

If your doctors suggest that you get a certain test, ask if the result will truly help determine your care. Sometimes I had a test done only to find out that the results would not affect my care. Ask your doctors to pause a moment and thoroughly assess just how critical a specific test is for you.

Some doctors may standardly suggest more tests than other doctors. It might have to do with the type of incentive a doctor is getting from an insurance carrier. Some insurance carriers might reward doctors for performing more tests; other might reward those doctors who perform fewer tests. It depends upon the type of insurance plan you have. Some doctors might willingly conduct tests to avoid lawsuits. You need to approach your doctors about the necessity of tests that they suggest.

Be aware that tests might work against you for disability purposes.

A negative test result can sometimes work against you. Your doctor, for example, may know that your condition has only a small chance of showing up on a MRI or other test. Just because it does not show up, however, does not necessarily mean you do not have that ailment. Disability reviewers can then hold that against you. You have to weigh all of these factors to determine how worthwhile a test is.

Tests and Insurance Coverage

If your doctors suggest that you get testing done in their offices, and that you also do another test at home, don't assume that the insurance company pays for all the testing at the same coinsurance level.

One of my doctors is contracted with my medical insurance carrier. That means my overall costs will not be as high as if I go to a doctor who is not contracted with my insurance carrier. My doctor ordered a test that I was to do in his office, and another that I would do at home. The home test involved my wearing a monitor. I called my insurance company to see how the testing would be paid. The company that provides the monitor is not contracted with my insurance company. That meant that I could end

up having to pay a few thousand dollars for the use of the monitor at home. The test that was being done in the office, and the
interpretation of the test, was covered at a contracted rate. This
is an example of why it's critical that patients always check how
procedures, visits, tests, and other medical care will be paid.

❦❧❦❧

The Consequences
of Clerical Errors

Clerical Errors

Don't underestimate the power of clerical errors.

Seemingly small clerical errors can turn into major problems for patients. Some errors even result in life-threatening situations.

Several years ago, I told my doctor I was concerned about my weight loss of ten pounds. He glanced at my chart and said not to worry. I thought it was strange that he was not concerned. I peeked at my chart when he left the room to see if the nurse who weighed me had written down the correct weight. She had put down that I weighed ninety-three pounds instead of eighty-three. I told the nurse about the error. She apologized and said that, subconsciously, she probably could not have imagined anyone weighing so little.

Another time, one of my doctors told me to skip a physical therapy appointment before I saw him. He thought it would help him to better assess my back problem. I did what he instructed. When I arrived at his office for my appointment, his receptionist said that I did not have an appointment that day. I showed her the card on which their office had written down the appointment time. I had even confirmed the appointment two days ago, but they still would not see me. I was surprised, because other offices I go to would have tried to fit me in.

Another time, I was told to perform a test at home. I mailed the completed test to the lab, only to find out that the lab discarded it because I had been given an expired test kit. I had to get another kit and repeat the test. I informed my doctor of the old expiration date, and I suggested that her office check for such things in the future. Patients, too, should check the expiration dates.

I once caught an error in which the wrong foot was marked on the paperwork for my surgery. You need to be on guard for such errors.

One of the worst mishaps was the day of my hysterectomy. Prior to surgery, I was brought to a large room to wait for the doctor. Apparently, someone did not place me in the appropriate area, so the doctor had trouble locating me. Being the great doctor that he is, he spent a lot of time trying to find me. He told me that he almost gave up searching for me. That surgery, which was necessary because I had ovarian cancer, had required major fasting and courage on my part. It would have been devastating to me if it had been canceled.

A doctor once told me to buy a specific over-the-counter product to put in my eye. After searching endlessly in the drugstore for it, I finally asked the pharmacist where I could locate it. The pharmacist told me that I was lucky they didn't have it in stock. He said that had I put it in my eye, it most likely would have caused me to go blind. Prior to going to the store, my instincts urged me to ask my eye doctor's opinion of the product. I should have listened to my instincts.

I once had a dental CAT scan. I was put in a room separate from where the technicians were. They said they would be talking to me through a sound system and that I should follow their directions. I could see their mouths moving, but there was no sound. Apparently, they had forgotten to turn on the sound system. The test had to be redone because I turned my head the wrong way. That could have been avoided had they adequately checked the sound system before beginning the test.

A dentist prescribed a medication for me to take prior to a dental procedure. The quantity of pills that I was supposed to take seemed high, so I immediately called him. He agreed that he mistakenly indicated a much higher amount than I should take for my size and weight. That "clerical" error in medication could have had severe consequences for me.

When a homeopathic doctor gave me a remedy, he wrote out instructions on how to take it. I was told to take a certain number of drops twice a day for five days, and then take two drops. I thought that meant that I should completely stop the medicine after the two drops. He meant that I should take two drops twice a day until I saw him next. I almost called him to question the instructions, but didn't because some of my doctors had recently told me I was asking too many questions. I was afraid the homeo-pathic doctor would also get irritated by my questions. Looking back, I realize I should have called him. This example shows how doctors must be very specific when writing out instructions, as well as how important it is for a patient to call the doctor if any-thing seems amiss.

My friend was scheduled for an endoscopic procedure. After he arrived at the testing facility, he was sent home because he had not stopped taking one of his medications five days prior to the test. No one had previously informed him that he should stop the medicine. The test had to be rescheduled.

Prior to getting MRI tests, I call facilities to be sure they have received all of the information from my doctor. A doctor once told me that I must have an injection with contrast dye during my MRI test. When I arrived at the facility, they said that the doctor had not authorized the contrast. I had to wait until they resolved it.

If your doctor's office says they will send something to another one of your doctors, check to be sure that doctor received it. Sometimes things get lost in the mail. Items also get lost in piles of papers on desks. On several occasions, I've had to ask recep-tionists to resend things.

Don't assume that your insurance carrier will pay for hospital neglect.

Hospital-acquired infections are costly. I've read that Medicare and some insurance companies will not pay for certain conditions that are due to medical errors in hospitals.[39] Careless errors in hospitals can cost you not only in terms of your health, but also your wallet.

Don't assume that your insurance carrier's website is always current.

Do not assume that information on your insurance carrier's web-site is always current and includes all the details of your insurance plan. Some claim representatives told me that their employer's website was not current, and did not list all the details of my ben-efits. I call the claim office when I need to know how something will be paid. You might, however, call the claim office and still be given the wrong information.

I called my dental claim office once to get some information. They told me I had a particular dental plan and that it was currently effective. I knew that plan had expired the prior year. I prefer calling, versus reviewing benefits online, because at least I can say that a claim representative had given me the information. I feel they will be less likely to hold that against me if something goes wrong in the payment process.

Take precautions to prevent your own clerical errors. Complete forms neatly and accurately. Be honest with your doctors, and keep them informed of changes in your medication or condition.

Some doctors told me I'm too particular and compulsive about my care. I don't expect them to like my persistence. Don't let unfair comments distract you from getting the care you deserve.

※※※※

Surgeries, Surveys, Rooms

Procedures

Keep a copy of all paperwork that you completed for surgical procedures, and bring a copy to the surgical center.

You will have paperwork to complete prior to your surgery, and will most likely have to get pre-admission testing. I suggest keeping a copy of that paperwork and bringing it with you to your surgery. My paperwork usually had to be hunted down when I got to surgical centers. I got so fed up with my paperwork being lost at a particular facility that I hand delivered it the day before my surgery. To my surprise, the facility still lost it. Fortunately, I had brought a copy with me on the day of the surgery. Usually, you will also need to sign papers at the facility on the day of your surgery.

Be sure you are weighed prior to surgery and certain tests.

I think all facilities should weigh patients on their day of surgery. My weight was taken just before surgeries on only a few occasions. Usually, anesthesiologists just asked me what I weighed. I realize weight is taken during pre-admission testing, but that could have been up to thirty days ago. I didn't have a scale at home, and even if I did, I question how accurate home scales are. Most people probably do not have much of a weight change between pre-admission testing and surgery. Those with anorexia, bulimia, and other medical conditions, however, might have a sudden change in their weight.

Prior to entering the surgical room for one of my surgeries, I asked the nurse to weigh me. It was during a time when my weight was fluctuating quite a bit. I was laughed at and told I could go down the hall to weigh myself. I went down the hall only to find a broken scale.

Prior to my bone density tests, my weight was not always taken by the testing facilities. Weight is important in the analysis of that test. One technician said she would just use the weight from the prior year. I told her not to, since I was ten pounds lighter than the prior year. You have to watch out for carelessness. Such indifference may be due to the staff not wanting to take the time for certain tasks or because some people are not naturally detail-oriented. If you have any question as to whether a facility should be weighing you just before a test, ask your doctor ahead of time. If you know you should be weighed, and the technician is not offering to weigh you, speak up and insist on it.

Prior to my bone density test, I was instructed not to take calcium supplements or a multi-vitamin within twenty-four hours of the test. Ask the facility you go to what its guidelines are. If you are scheduled for a bone density test, ask your doctor if your left and right hips will be tested. Most facilities I went to tested the density of only one hip. If you want both hips tested, discuss it with your doctor. Ask your insurance carrier if it pays for testing both hips. Some technicians and doctors told me that it was not necessary to test both hips. I disagree with their belief. I think that significant differences in bone density can exist in a person's left hip versus their right hip.

Ask your doctor to send you a copy of your bone density report and images. One of the reports stated that my overall density was fairly good. When I looked at the report, however, I noticed two regions in my hip had a much lower density than the other regions of the hip. I think advancements need to be made in bone density testing and assessments.

If you have special medical needs, inform your doctor and the staff ahead of time.

If you need to be catheterized for a surgical procedure, check ahead of time to ensure that the facility has someone to do it. Most outpatient facilities that I went to did not have a nurse who knew how to insert a catheter, or they had just one nurse capable of the task. Be sure you are scheduled on a day the person who can meet your special needs will be available. I was surprised that one hospital I went to told me no one was available to catheterize me early in the morning.

Find out the days that your doctor performs surgery.

I avoid getting surgery on a Friday, if possible. I'm concerned that my doctor might not be available in the event that post-surgical issues arose over the weekend. I also like to avoid being admitted to a hospital on a weekend, because I think the care will be better Monday through Friday when a full staff is on duty.

Ask your doctors if they anticipate a shortage of your medication.

Drug shortages in hospitals have increased over the past few years.[40] Shortages have included chemotherapy drugs, heart medications, anesthetic drugs, and some syringes.[41] If your doctor suspects your medication will not be obtainable, ask about the potential consequences of taking another drug.

Second Opinions and Pre-Approvals

Get a second opinion for surgery.

If surgery is suggested, consider getting a second, or even third, opinion. You'll have to check with your insurance carrier to see if the extra opinions are covered. An insurance company might require that you get another opinion. I've found such mandatory requirements to be lessening over the years. Sometimes your doctor will give you the name of a specific physician to consult. I get concerned if they know each other. They may be hesitant to offer an opinion that is contrary that of their colleague. Occasionally, I will elect to keep the name of another doctor private. One doctor said that he could see, in the computer system, the names of other doctors that I had gone to at his facility.

Sometimes second opinions backfire. My doctor had requested an ultrasound test for me because he suspected an ovarian tumor. After seeing the test results, he didn't think that I had cancer. He said he was going to get another opinion from a doctor that he knew. I told him that I would also get a few more opinions. Thus, there were several opinions overall, and none of those doctors thought I had cancer. A laparoscopy was then done to break up my ovarian cyst. The biopsy showed that it was ovarian cancer. Unfortunately, the laparoscopy had caused the cancer to spread microscopically throughout my body.

Don't rely on your doctor's staff for pre-certifications and authorizations of treatments.

Some insurance plans require authorization for certain tests; other plans might not. Usually your physician's staff will coordinate necessary approvals for surgeries and treatments. You should check with your insurance company to be sure that your doctor's office has followed the correct guidelines. The doctor's office may find that intrusive, but remember that you are probably the one that will bear the financial burden for the claim. I often found that the appropriate procedures were not followed.

If you have multiple insurance carriers, be sure that they all are notified for pre-approvals. Most offices that I went to only notified two insurance carriers for pre-certification, ignoring my third carrier. If the first two had not fully paid for the procedure, I would have wanted my third insurance carrier to consider it.

Fasting Prior to Procedures

If you have trouble fasting or have medical conditions that would make fasting difficult, inform your doctor.

If you have concerns that fasting will be difficult for you, tell your doctor. Fasting can be particularly problematic for those with diabetes, hypoglycemia, and other medical conditions.

Most facilities will consider your medical conditions when determining what patients are taken first. It's been said that having the first surgery of the day may not work to your advantage. Some doctors think that getting the second or third surgical slot is better, because all of the kinks in the surgical team's coordination efforts and machines will have been worked out by then.[42]

Once, I had to fast two full days prior to a surgery. It was a very difficult fast. I had asked the appropriate staff at the hospital if I could come in early if I felt weak. The hospital assured me that would not be a problem. When I awoke the morning of the surgery, I felt like I was going to pass out. My husband drove me to the facility early. When I arrived, they gave me a hard time about arriving so early. They finally put me in a room, and I overheard a nurse say, "I knew she'd do this." I was very weak, and I found her remark to be rude. I later found out the weakness was due to my blood pressure having dropped so low.

Doctors need to be very specific when they are talking to their patients about fasting. If you take medication, ask your doctor if you should take it the morning of the surgery. Sometimes you may be told not to take medication. It is critical that you follow your doctor's instructions.

My father-in-law thought that fasting meant not to eat his usual portion of food, so he ate a piece of toast prior to his surgery. He was sent home from the hospital, and the surgery had to be rescheduled.

I have a little trick that makes fasting easier for me. I normally eat breakfast around five o'clock in the morning. Suppose I am scheduled for a blood test at eight o'clock in the morning. A few weeks before my procedure, I'll eat my breakfast a little bit later each day until I get used to eating at eight o'clock. That way, fasting until eight o'clock is not such a shock to my body. I realize that gradually increasing time between meals could be difficult for some people who are required to take medications at a certain time with food. Check with your doctor to see if this might be a good system for you.

Are You Considered Inpatient or Outpatient?

If you are a patient in a hospital, be aware that you might be considered to be outpatient.

If you have Medicare and are in a hospital for more than a few hours, ask the hospital if you are considered to have inpatient or outpatient status.[43] The hospital must receive an order from your doctor to formally admit you as an inpatient.[44] The day prior to your discharge is considered to be your last inpatient day.[45] Your hospital status will determine how much your insurance will cover for certain services.

Even if you don't have Medicare, ask your insurance company about your hospital status. It's good to know how payments should be made, so you can be sure you are being billed correctly. It's also good to make a family member aware of status issues in case you are admitted to a hospital on an emergency basis and are unable to obtain that information on your own.

Get Supplies Prior to Your Surgery

Prior to your day of surgery, get all the after-care supplies that you can.

If you've had the same surgery before, you might recall that some items are helpful to have on hand. I bought special bandages and medical tape that I knew I'd need after my foot surgeries. I also set up my bed ahead of time with extra pillows to elevate my legs. I put a portable toilet in my bedroom. I prepared all the ice that I'd need to reduce swelling in my feet. I got the thermometer out in case I developed a fever, and I charged my cell phone. I made sure that my husband knew where to locate my will, living will, health directives, and list of medications and allergies. I even packed a small suitcase in the event I had to stay overnight at the hospital.

It would be great if doctors had designated staff persons to go over post-operative issues with patients prior to their surgery. My experience has been that doctors do not give enough time or support to help a patient assess pre-operative or post-operative care. I appreciate a doctor who gives me a heads-up as to what sensations or conditions are normal after a specific surgery.

After surgery, your doctor might give you a prescription for pain-relief medication. Most of us probably won't feel up to going to a drugstore to fill a prescription right after being released from the surgical center. If you send a friend or family member to fill your prescription, that person may be the very person you need to be with you at home. On occasion, the drugstore may have to order the medicine. Some practitioners gave me the prescriptions ahead of time. Most of the surgeons that my husband and I have had, however, would not give us the prescription until after our procedures. This is understandable, as sometimes the doctor really does not know what you will need until after the surgery is done. Perhaps there are legal ramifications, too.

If necessary, consider purchasing special clothing that is easier to get on and off. Some stores offer nightgowns that will fully open in the front or side, making it easier to get them on and off. They might also offer shirts that you can open and close via Velcro instead of buttons. Some stores sell special shoes for people with edema. Such clothing can be very beneficial to those in a nursing home or at home recuperating from surgery. You will find several online sites that offer a variety of special clothing. Some places will imprint your name in clothing so that it's less likely your clothing will get lost at a medical facility.

Will you be using a wheelchair after surgery? If so, consider how you will get into your house. I purchased a portable wheelchair ramp that fit over the step to my house.

Will you need to use crutches after surgery? If you think it will be difficult for you to use crutches, ask your doctor if it could benefit you to sometimes use a knee walker instead. If your surgery is not urgently needed, ask your doctor if you can practice using crutches a few months prior to the surgery. Make sure your crutches are adjusted to the appropriate height.

I think most doctors don't realize how much time it takes patients to prepare for surgery. My situation was such that I had to coordinate my physical therapy with when I was to receive surgery. Juggling everything can require a lot of upfront work for patients and their families. A patient may also have to arrange for rides or find a babysitter for their children. A spouse may need to plan for time off from work. If patients won't be able to drive for a while, they may need to get groceries ahead of time. It is a very hectic time for patients and their families.

Latex Allergy

If you have an allergy to latex, make sure your practitioners are using non-latex gloves when treating you.

I develop skin irritations to latex if used for extended times. When I informed the nurses and doctors of this, they told me to list latex as an allergy so the medical staff would wear latex-free gloves. The problem is that the facilities may not have them in stock. I once asked a nurse why latex-free gloves are so scarce around offices. She told me it's because they are expensive and that facilities want their employees to avoid using them unless absolutely necessary. A nurse once tried to convince me that I didn't react to latex because she could not locate any latex-free gloves in the room. When I insisted that I did, she searched for them in another part of the building.

Risks of Surgery

Find out the risks of the surgery prior to the day of surgery.

Sometimes I hadn't seen the papers that explain the risks of the surgery until I arrived at the surgical center. I am usually tired and weak then from having fasted and not at my best intellectually. I think all patients should be shown this information ahead of time. It gives patients time to think about what risks they may not want to take. After reading the risks, you may have more questions for your doctor. The same holds true for undergoing any medical test. I think doctors should thoroughly go over risks during an office visit. I've asked some doctors about specific risks and was told I did not have to be concerned about those issues. When I was presented with surgical forms to sign, those items were listed as risks. Patients need to demand more from their doctors regarding this issue. Our bodies, not theirs, will be affected.

Ask your doctor if you will be placed in a steep Trendelenburg position during surgery, which is a head-down position that can increase pressure on the back of the optic nerve and cause permanent blindness.[46] The position is most common in robotic surgeries or lengthy laparoscopic procedures, and some hospitals periodically take patients out of the head-down position or administer eye drops to reduce pressure.[47] Ask the hospital, where you will have surgery, if it takes precautions against steep head-down positions.

Washing Hands and Sterilizing Instruments

Ask the surgical team if they have washed and scrubbed their hands.

You have to hope that your doctors are washing their hands between patients. Equally important, patients should wash their hands when warranted. I don't like it when doctors shake my hand during the flu season. If you are having surgery, certainly the surgeon and others helping with the surgery should be scrubbing and washing their hands. It's not a bad idea to check to be sure they all have done this. If you do, be prepared that some doctors and staff may think that you are over-reacting.

It's also important to ask your doctors if they sterilized their surgical instruments.

July Surgeries

If your surgery is not urgent, ask your doctor the best time of year for you to have surgery.

A surgeon once told me to avoid surgery in July. When I asked him why, he responded that residents are in training at that time, and thus more errors are likely. Another doctor told me that issue was controversial. I have read that there is a 10 percent hike in fatalities at teaching hospitals in July due to medication errors.[48] I had surgery in July, before knowing it might even be a concern. Fortunately, all went well, and I experienced no problems during the procedure. You certainly don't want to postpone a surgery that your doctor feels is urgent. Discuss any concerns about the timing of your surgery with your doctor.

You doctor might prefer that you have surgery at a certain time of the year. For example, if you have circulation problems, the doctor might prefer that you have the surgery in the summer when it's warm out.

Patients' Rooms

Ask your visitors to keep an eye out for spoiled food and dirty personal items.

If you have to undergo a procedure that may also require extended care in a facility, there are some things you should tell your family members, or other visitors, to watch out for. For instance, they should inform the nurses if they notice that untouched food and beverages brought to you earlier in the day are still sitting by your bedside later in the day. You don't want to eat food several hours after it was brought to you and get ill because it sat too long at room temperature. It's also important that visitors report an untouched beverage, because a nurse may have added medication to it. If you wear glasses, ask your visitors to clean them if you can't. Ask visitors to place items that you are allowed to use, such as a remote control, within your reach.

When you are recovering, you may be groggy and not alert enough to spot these issues the way your visitor easily can. I recently read that Connecticut state health regulators found that many patients at a specific nursing home were not even given their medications.[49] This shows how important it is that you have someone watching out for you.

If you have a catheter in while you are at the facility, ask your spouse or significant other to take a peek to be sure the bag is not full or near full. That is, of course, if you have discussed that task in advance and your visitor is comfortable with it. The visitor should not touch the catheter or move it around. I'm speaking of this in the sense of just glancing to see if the bag is full. I had a catheter in during my hysterectomy, and the nurse was usually very good about coming in to check the bag. One day, however, she was so busy that she was not able to get to the room as frequently. When I noticed that the bag was nearly full, I shouted out until a nurse finally heard me and came in. If the bag fills up and is not emptied, it can cause critical problems for the patient. With the shortage of nurses in some facilities, you have to hope nurses are able to come in soon enough to check the bags in a timely manner.

Your visitors should ask the facility what type of gifts can be brought into your room.

Flowers can be uplifting, but they can become a burden to patients and caregivers. Real flowers usually die quickly and their leaves wither and fall. They can also emit an odor if the water has not been changed. It can become a hassle to have to keep cleaning the vase out. Visitors should not bring in a plant that has poisonous berries on it. I prefer artificial flowers for these reasons. Flowers can also cause a lot of clutter on a patient's table. If you anticipate that these may be issues for you, politely inform close friends and family members that you prefer not to receive flowers. You can suggest plants, which usually require less care. It can be awkward talking to others about gifts, but if you know that your parents or siblings are bound to bring you something, it's worth discussing this with them ahead of time.

Likewise, if you are visiting a patient sometime, keep these things in mind. If you want to bring an edible gift to your friend or loved one, get permission from the facility. You should ask the nurse about any item you want to bring into a patient's room. There may be strict guidelines, and for good reasons.

I once brought a helium balloon to a friend in the hospice area, not knowing balloons were not allowed. It was a giant Tweety Bird balloon, which I later found out became loose during the night. Apparently, it was hovering around the room until a nurse spotted it and took it away. It was rather humorous, but not the best of circumstances for the patient. I am very thankful that it did not get caught in my friend's oxygen machine.

If you are recuperating from surgery at home, use caution when taking flowers from a delivery person. Someone sent me a very large bouquet of flowers in a vase after my hysterectomy. I almost grabbed the vase from the delivery person. She was very smart and asked me if I had just had surgery. She must have noticed the card telling me to get well. I suddenly remembered that I was not supposed to lift anything heavy for six weeks. I was so grateful that the delivery person was attentive. If you are sending flowers to someone who had surgery, consider ordering an arrangement that is not too heavy.

Surgical Discharge Instructions

If you find differences between the hospital discharge instructions and those from your doctor, ask your doctor and the facility which instructions you should follow.

Each time I had surgery, I was given conflicting discharge instructions. Facilities would give me one set of instructions and my doctors another. They never matched up 100 percent in terms of how long to ice an area, how high to raise a leg, or how frequently to change a bandage. I questioned conflicting discharge instructions after all of my surgeries. Nurses would then have to locate the doctors to ask which set of instructions I should follow.

The nurses seemed frustrated that I had asked because it was taking them time to find the doctor. I felt like the facility and doctor didn't want me to notice the differences. I realize that they were just following their own procedures, but contradicting instructions are confusing to patients. Also, if you develop post-surgical problems, someone could say you did not follow the proper guidelines if you don't question the conflicting instructions.

Surveys

Remain anonymous when completing surveys.

After one of my surgeries, I was asked to complete a survey. I mentioned it would be helpful if patients could get their prescriptions prior to their surgical procedure. I also noted on the survey that I had overheard another patient bring this up while I was in the recovery room. I admit I hesitated putting that in the survey, as I had no business in that person's affairs. After over-hearing the other patient, I wanted the facility to know that others felt the same way. I thought it would be helpful for the facility to see it from a patient's viewpoint.

Unfortunately, the survey came back to haunt me. My doctor later told me that the facility did not know if they wanted me as a patient anymore, due to my survey response. I was surprised because I was very tactful in my approach. My aim was to help patients in such a situation. I also didn't think it was fair that my survey comments were being held against me.

You might be asked to complete surveys over the phone. I think the ones over the phone are too general to give an accurate assessment. They can lock you into an answer that you don't necessarily agree with.

Pets in Patient Rooms

If you don't want pets around you, inform the staff.

Many people in nursing homes or extended care facilities do not desire to have pets around them. Some people are uncomfortable around animals and may be agitated by them. Some facilities think pets are great for companionship. Pets can be wonderful for those who find them comforting but not for those who don't. Pets can be hazardous for those with walking impairments who have to worry about tripping over a cat or dog. Perhaps there could be a special room with pets where those who want to be around them could periodically stop in. You have to be concerned with those who have allergies to pets. You also don't want a patient with dementia to accidentally harm a pet. State laws vary regarding pets in nursing homes.

Use caution around your home if you have pets.

You need to consider the issue of pets around your home, too. Many with balance problems can easily fall by tripping over a small pet or from a large dog bumping into them. It may sound silly to someone in good physical shape, but to a frail person this can easily trigger a fall or injury.

Claims, Medical Equipment, Physical Therapy

How to Avoid Claim Problems

Keep track of phone conversations and who you spoke with regarding insurance claims.

If you have a very important phone discussion with a claims representative, it's helpful to write that person a letter to confirm the discussion. I had a critical conversation with my insurance company regarding a legal matter. I not only wrote my own letter to the person I talked to, but I also asked that he write one to me. To my surprise, he sent me a letter confirming the details of the conversation. Thank goodness I saved the letter; a few years later, the same issue arose again. The insurance representative who originally handled the issue said that he had never written me about the subject. That letter helped me to prove that he had previously written me, and it helped me settle the issue. This has happened to me on more than one occasion.

Be persistent to get accurate information from claims specialists.

A pet peeve of mine is being rushed on the phone by a claims specialist. I don't fault the claims specialists, because it's most likely the rules under which they have to operate. They may be required to complete calls within a certain timeframe.

I ask the person who answers what their name is. Most claims representatives I talked to would not give me their last names, but I can often get them to at least give me the initials of their last names. I've discovered a crafty way to get their names or initials of their last names. As soon as they ask me my name, I tell them. Then, I cut into the conversation and ask for their names. If they give me a hard time I say, "Just as you need my last name for certain reasons, I need your last name for my reasons." It puts them on the spot. Sometimes a person will tell me they are the only person working there with their first name, so they don't think it's necessary to say their last name. If you have to call the company back months later, it can get confusing if a newly hired person also has that same first name. Ask representatives to identify the city and state of the claim office in which they work. If you have to call back for the same issue, you most likely will be asked who you previously spoke to and where they work.

Be aware of customer service specialists who give you hazy answers. You can usually tell if they do not sound confident in their answer. If the representatives use words like, "I think," "probably," or "don't worry," they may not be sure of what they are telling you. You have to be assertive and ask if they are certain about their answer. They will probably say no and switch you to someone else who can answer your question. If you just go along with their first responses, you may never get the correct answer.

I have had some excellent customer service representatives, as well as those who seem to pretend to know what they are saying. I've done experiments in which I've called the same claims office with the same question several times, and gotten several different answers. Some claims representatives told me they never received my claims, even though other representatives previously assured me my claims were there. Some claims representatives have told me they can't see all the information on the screen. Nonetheless, when I've asked them to hunt around more, they usually found the claims. One claims representative told me a certain procedure was covered at 100 percent coinsurance. A few days later, however, a different claim representative told me the procedure is paid at 80 percent coinsurance, subject to the deductible.

If a claims representative is going to transfer you to someone else, get the name of the person, the department, and the phone number of who they are transferring you to in case you get disconnected. The claims person should be telling you that, but often they don't.

Be sure the claims person hears and absorbs what you say during a conversation. I was surprised by the number of times I said something, and a minute later, the person asked me a question to which I had already given an answer. I might have, for example, just stated my name and phone number. Right after that, the representative asked for my phone number. I think the claims representatives are looking at a screen and are so focused on answering each item in a specific order that they do not hear when you throw something extra in. If they ask you for your name, say only your name and nothing else. Take it one step at a time.

Make copies of claims that you submit yourself. Check claim statements for accuracy.

Check the explanation of benefits that you receive from your insurance company. The majority that I received for out-of-network claims had errors. I found incorrect dates of services and incorrect procedures listed. Claims of other people were sent to me by mistake. You want to be sure the deductible is being applied correctly and that you are getting the payment you deserve. I saved myself thousands of dollars by catching errors.

Most offices will submit claims for you. (If Medicare is your primary provider, I believe the doctor's office is required to submit claims for you). Most offices will submit claims electronically. Usually electronic processing is the most efficient way, as long as an office is handling your claims correctly. I sometimes choose to submit my own claims because I know I will send them to the correct insurance carrier. I have multiple insurance carriers, and some offices have mistakenly sent my claims to my secondary or tertiary carrier first, instead of to my primary insurance carrier. I then have to call my doctors' offices to tell them they submitted it to the wrong carrier. They always tell me they will correct it, but many times offices still continued to submit it to the wrong carrier. One office told me they did not have all of my insurance information even though I had given it to them on several occasions.

I also consider submitting my own claims if the office had many mix-ups with my claims in the past. If you submit your own claims, make a copy of every page you submit. Many of my claims were lost at insurance companies. My husband once had to fax the same claim twelve times before the insurance company said it received it, despite the fax machine acknowledging an acceptable transmission. For claims of utmost importance that you submit on your own, I suggest sending them via certified mail and requesting a return receipt. That way, someone has to sign that they received it, and you have proof. Definitely use some type of tracking method.

Many times, I had paid for a service upfront and filled out the claim form indicating that remittance should be sent to me and not the facility. I did that by not checking the assignment box on the claim form. Mistakenly, the insurance company would often send the check to the doctor's office anyway. Then I had to wait for the doctor to either sign the check over to me or return it to the insurance company for reprocessing. It was not uncommon for me to wait nearly a year to get my money.

You might accidentally receive money that you do not deserve from a claim office. I received thousands of dollars of duplicate checks and returned all of them. It would be nice to have the extra money, but obviously, you must be truthful. Call the insurance company to see how they want you to return the money and who you should send it to. Some places told me to rip up the check. Other places wanted me to return the check to them as long as I hadn't signed it yet.

Examine bills carefully.

If you get a bill from your doctor's office, check it for accuracy. If you have lots of doctor visits, keep a log of your claim history. I've found incorrect dates of service, incorrect charges, and duplicate charges on doctors' bills. Examine the accuracy of your hospital statements too.

Sometimes I received checks from my insurance carrier that did not state the provider. I couldn't figure out why I was being sent money, since I didn't pay for any services that year. In one situation, the check was for a claim from three years ago. Apparently, during an audit, it was discovered that I was owed money. If you receive a check for which no date of service is listed, call the claim office to find out the specifics. That way, you can be sure you really deserve the check before you cash it.

Some practitioners wanted to apply all of the money that they owed me to my next visit. Sometimes I was not going to come into the office for another six months. I had money due from many offices, and it all added up. It didn't seem fair that I should have to wait so long for my money. At times, I had more than $500 due to me from multiple offices, and I was not getting interest on the money while I waited. You need to be assertive to get the money you deserve, and to receive it in a timely manner. When money was applied to future visits, it became confusing for claim and tax purposes.

Understand that an insurance company may later deny a service it once approved.

Don't think that just because you received reimbursement for a claim, the insurance company won't try to get the money back later. It happened to me. For several years, an insurance company had paid for my physical therapy. They later tried to recover more than $10,000 from me for physical therapy expenses. They said they should not have paid it. I was shocked, since I had spoken with the supervisor and claims representatives many times about my claims. Not once did anyone suggest that checks were sent to me in error. I had even talked to the supervisor a few weeks prior to getting notification that the company wanted money back. During that time, the supervisor and I even discussed money that was still owed to me, and I was told my physical therapy was covered. Furthermore, they sent me checks for reimbursement after those discussions. I had to appeal the entire issue, and I won on the second appeal.

Insurance Appeals

Don't give up if your first appeal is denied.

Another stress can be the appeals process for insurance claims. You may have had several medical visits that your insurance company paid for, but it might later notify you that coverage will stop because it thinks the care is no longer necessary. Or, you may find your insurance carrier does not want to pay for a service from the start. An insurance company may know that it already paid you for a service, but it might later try to recoup claim payments. Check with your medical insurance carrier to find out what your rights are regarding the appeal process.

To appeal, you will not only have to do so within certain time parameters, but you will have to send evidence to support your appeal. It's helpful to get a letter from your doctor to support your appeal. Some doctors will charge you for the letter. My doctors' fees ranged from no charge to seventy-five dollars per letter. Your insurance company, once having reviewed your appeal, may still determine that the treatment is not covered. You will usually be allowed another chance to appeal as long as you submit new supporting evidence. Take advantage of that. None of my appeals won the first time around, but they always did the second time. You might need to get an updated letter from your doctor or an attorney to support your second appeal.

Your insurance carrier might have a medical consultant review your first appeal. If that person determined that you should not receive benefits, ask the insurance company to send you a copy of the consultant's notes. This will allow you to see the specifics of why your appeal was denied. This information will be helpful to you if you are writing a second appeal.

My insurance company merely sent me a standard letter stating that my first appeal was denied because they thought the care was not necessary. Once I got the consultant's notes, however, I was able to see there was much more to it than that. Part of the reason I was denied benefits for one of my claims was that my doctor had not filled out a certain form. Neither I, nor my doctor, had previously been sent the form or been told it was needed. I requested that the insurance company send my doctor the form. He completed it, and I won the appeal.

Don't give up too easily if you feel you deserve benefits that the insurance company denied. The insurer most likely wants you to give up, so it won't have to pay those benefits.

Answering Services

Learn the tricks of answering systems.

A message on an answering system might say that you are calling during a busy time and suggest you call back later. Furthermore, it might tell you the estimated wait time. My calls were usually taken within a few minutes even when answering systems said I would have a long wait. I don't know if offices are hoping that callers hang up, thinking they will have to wait too long, or if the systems aren't good at estimating wait times.

One of my pet peeves is an answering system telling people to please call back when the office is open, when it's already well beyond the opening time.

Some offices have a message on the answering machine that tells you to hold for the next representative. After you hold for an excessively long time, however, you realize they are not even open yet. I thought an office opened at seven o'clock in the morning and made my call soon after that. After holding for a long time, I suddenly remembered that they were not open until eight o'clock. The machine kept telling me to hold for the next representative, which gave me the impression someone would be coming to the phone fairly soon. The reality was that no one was even around for almost a full hour. The message should have said that they are closed and mentioned when they reopen.

Some offices are open earlier than they take phone calls. I realize they most likely have a legitimate reason for this. Many places have meetings first thing in the morning. If an office tells you they open at nine o'clock, don't be surprised if they don't start picking up the phone until nine thirty or later.

Medical Equipment

Make sure you know how to use medical equipment properly before taking it home.

If your doctor provides you with rental equipment to take home, ask the staff to assure you that it's in good working condition and if the programs for the machine are set correctly. I was given a machine to use at home and tried it at the settings as instructed. Something did not feel right. I called my doctor's assistant who still thought the settings were okay. I then called the manufacturer of the machine, and I found out that the doctor's office didn't adjust the settings correctly. They had set the machine for the wrong ailment. If your doctor's office insists that they have handled things correctly, but you feel that something is amiss, consider calling the manufacturer yourself like I did. If they agree that something is not right, inform your doctor. Your doctor's assistants may not have been aware of certain aspects of the equipment, or they may not have been adequately trained.

At another facility, I received rental equipment that worked fine, but I wasn't given adequate training on how to use it. That resulted in my having to make several calls to the manufacturer to learn more about the meaning of the various controls.

If you leave the hospital with crutches, be sure you know how to use them. Most facilities I went to were fairly good about instructing me in this regard. I wish they also had stairs to practice on, though. It takes time to learn the proper way to go up and down steps with crutches. This also holds true for canes. Using crutches, wheelchairs, or canes incorrectly can cause you a lot more damage.

It's also important that you are given the proper size device for your height and weight. I made the mistake of trying to go down a sidewalk curb in a wheelchair that was too small for me. I almost flipped over. Don't think you can get into any wheelchair and safely navigate around in it, especially if attempting curbs or slopes.

If you need to buy a motorized scooter or wheelchair, check with your insurance company to see if it will cover the costs. The insurance company may have restrictions on the type it will consider. Prior to purchasing a scooter or motorized wheelchair to be used outside, contact your local police department to learn the rules that apply to using it in your town. Some towns might require that a scooter be capable of specific minimum or maximum speed limits for outside usage. There might also be regulations for motorized wheelchairs.

I often wonder if those who designed some of our medical supplies ever used them, because many are of such poor design. Have you ever used a product that adds extra height to a toilet seat? They are often too thick and too high. Manufacturers should design toilets that can easily be raised or lowered to various heights.

Physical Therapy Exercises

Ask your physical therapist if you can get a home-based program.
Always do your exercises in the proper form, to avoid injury.

If you are receiving physical therapy, you may eventually be able to get a home-based exercise program. Home programs can save you a lot of money. You must take the initiative to do your exercises, and you must be certain you are doing them correctly. Doing them incorrectly can cause more harm. Be sure your therapist is closely watching you when you do exercises in the office. This will ensure that you are doing them properly. You might even find it helpful to take notes on how to do them. That way, you can clearly remember how to do the exercises when you get home.

If you think you are being given too many exercises at once, tell your therapist. I found that I did best by learning just a few exercises at a time. The physical therapist may have a reason, however, for giving you several exercises at once.

To my disappointment, I've been in some physical therapy facilities where the therapists are given too many clients at one time. Those offices are like a production facility. The therapists at those facilities often shout out instructions across the room instead of standing by clients and carefully watching them. The focus for each patient is not there the way it should be. Some physical therapists watched the television in the treatment room more than they watched their patients.

I am incredibly thankful for my physical therapist. I have some treatments at the office, but I also have an exercise program that I do at home. The facility I go to offers private rooms, which I really like.

Wear comfortable clothing. Some physical therapy offices do not provide a gown to wear. If you wear clothing that restricts your movements, it will be difficult to perform exercises.

Orthotics

Take care in selecting the shoes in which your orthotics will go.

Orthotic inserts for shoes can help you attain the proper gait. You can buy them over-the-counter, but the ones that are custom-made are often the best, since they are made specifically for your own feet. If you want to get an assessment for orthotics, see a podiatrist or physical therapist. Unfortunately, very few of my podiatrists were concerned with how the orthotics would fit in my shoes. I would receive great orthotics, but once in my shoes, they felt uncomfortable. That was because my shoes were not deep enough to accommodate the orthotic, or because my shoes were designed in a way that threw off the angle of the orthotic.

Orthotics with postings on them can correct your feet from excessively rolling outwards (supination) or inwards (pronation). Many shoes are automatically made to accommodate pronation. A few are made to accommodate supination. If you then put an orthotic made for pronation in a shoe that is already made for pronation, your orthotic won't function as it should. The same goes for supination. My physical therapist was excellent regarding this, and she always encouraged me to buy shoes that were rather basic and not already designed for pronation or supination. You also have to watch how the heels of your shoes wear over time, because that can also affect your gait.

Some foot doctors sell shoes in their office that are specifically designed for use with orthotics. I long for the day when we can get custom-made shoes on the spot. After all, no two feet are alike.

Light and Temperature

While getting physical therapy, a massage, or other treatment in a private room, ask the practitioner if they will adjust the temperature and lighting to your needs. Also take into account the practitioner's preferences.

Is the temperature and lighting of a treatment room important to you? I love a lot of light in a room. I had to laugh when a physical therapist, who I had never met before, saw me sitting in a brightly lit room. She apologized for the room not being dim. She laughed when I told her that I loved the brightness. If you are getting physical therapy or other treatment in a private room, ask the practitioner to adjust the lights to your liking. If a window is open and it's too cold for you, ask if they will close it. You can even request a blanket.

Be considerate of the practitioner's needs, too, and be sure they can work comfortably in the lighting and temperature that you request.

Pain Scales and Pain Management

Pain Scales and Pain Ratings

If you don't think the pain scale of 1 to 10 is an effective method to rate your pain, tell your practitioner.

Your practitioner might ask you to rate your pain on a scale of 1 to 10. (Some pain scales range from 0 to 10.) I found this very hard to do for fibromyalgia and interstitial cystitis because the symptoms vary so much. I once had a torn Achilles tendon; that was easy to rate because there was a steady progression of healing. I think a scale of 1 to 10 is a poor tool for assessing chronic conditions whose symptoms are variable. I usually fill the rating form out by saying the intensity of pain changes throughout the day. Sometimes I might write, for example, that my pain varies from a 2 to 8. Practitioners may not be happy about that, but it's the best I can offer.

There are other methods to rate pain, but most scales I've seen fail to adequately address chronic pain.

Our medical system needs a better way to describe and rate pain. For example, some people with urological conditions use the term "pain" to describe the sensation of pressure in the pelvic area. I, too, get that sensation, but I never thought of pressure as pain. I then realized that my doctors probably did not understand how much discomfort I was in because I told them I did not have pain.

My friend went to a hospital due to pressure in his chest. The doctors asked him if he had pain, and he said no. Later, when the doctors found out that he had severe pressure, they wanted to know why he said he didn't have pain. He didn't define pressure as pain.

I am not discounting anyone's discomfort. Each individual feels sensations differently. I think of pain as what I have experienced when I broke a bone. I think of my other sensations as intense discomfort. Hospitals should put less focus on the word "pain" and more focus on a patient's description of what they feel, such as pressure, squeezing, itching, burning, or cramping.

It's acceptable to use the word pain in the sense of pain management, to some extent. It's sometimes a misleading term for an individual's specific discomfort, though. We need different types of scales and ratings for specific conditions.

Pain Management

Talk to your doctor about available pain management options.

If your pain or discomfort is severely interfering with your daily activities, ask your doctors if they can suggest treatments and facilities that can help you function better. Each person may respond to the treatments differently. I've talked to several people who were not helped by pain clinic techniques. I am not discounting pain clinics, as they offer a variety of pain management techniques and can truly help some people. Our society needs to examine pain management more thoroughly. I will share with you some of what I have tried and what others have told me they tried for relief.

Imagery and meditation helped me to deal with nausea from chemotherapy. The only practitioners that help to temporarily alleviate my back pain are chiropractors, osteopaths, and physical therapists. No other pain management techniques have helped me in that regard. Other people with back trouble told me they found relief through yoga and acupuncture. One person told me her back pain was temporarily relieved by trigger point injections.

Transcutaneous electrical nerve stimulation (TENS) units are options for some people. A TENS unit can temporarily block pain. There are numerous other electrical devices for various types of problems. Biofeedback can help you get control over some bodily functions. If you are very tense and holding your muscles very tightly, biofeedback can train you to realize when you have muscle tension and help you learn to relax the muscles. Biofeedback is used for various medical conditions.

Some people benefit from wearing magnets, which can lessen pain and inflammation. Seek the advice of a qualified medical professional if you want to try magnetic therapy.

Rolfing helped my fibromyalgia more than any other treatment. Rolfing involves manipulating connective tissue. The best way I can describe it is as a very deep tissue massage. It was uncomfortable while I was undergoing it, but afterwards I felt much better.

Some people might get help through hypnosis for some types of conditions. There are several medications that may help to lessen pain.

Discuss your diet with you doctor. Some foods cause inflammation in the body. Your doctor might suggest you see a nutritionist. Reducing inflammation may help lessen some types of pain.

Sometimes, doing something creative can help distract you from pain. I've discovered that when I'm engrossed in reading a good book or making crafts, I temporarily forget about my pain. Of course, if you are in severe pain, such tactics may not work.

Check with your doctor about any treatment you want to try, even if you don't need a prescription for the treatment. Check with your insurance carrier to see what treatments your insurance plan covers.

Disability and Attorneys

Employer and Social Security Disability

Be sure your doctors complete your disability forms accurately and thoroughly.

Many employers have disability benefits for their employees. Some employers offer both short and long-term disability plans. Sometimes employees are required to sign up for these plans within a certain time following initial employment, although some employers will automatically provide those benefits. If you are on long-term disability, you will receive paperwork and periodic reviews. Assuming you meet disability requirements, disability plans commonly pay for physical reasons up to age fifty-five, or even age sixty-five, if you had elected the extra benefit.

Most long-term disability plans require your doctor(s) to complete a form stating the nature and extent of your disability. Some of my doctors were more willing than others to complete forms. Some doctors have more knowledge about disability guidelines than other doctors. Many doctors find the process too time-consuming.

Disability reviewers give less credibility to some types of practitioners than others. For example, an orthopedist might be viewed more highly than a chiropractor. In my case, reviewers did not give much credibility to my physical therapists. I found this unfair because physical therapists have helped me tremendously over the years.

Sometimes an employer disability plan requires that you to go to an independent medical consultant for an examination. This may help your employer determine whether you meet disability requirements. The consultant I was sent to had a bias against chiropractors, and he told me not to discuss chiropractic care in his office. If you think you are not being given a fair exam, inform your insurance carrier or whoever initially set up your exam.

Once you are on long-term disability, you will periodically receive a form to complete. You will have to complete one section of the form, and your doctor will have to complete the remaining sections. Usually the form will ask what your current activities of daily living are and if you want to participate in a rehabilitation program. Set up an appointment with your doctor to discuss the form. Ask your doctor to give you an updated assessment before he or she completes the form. Tell your doctor what you are currently capable of doing in terms of daily activities. For example, the form might ask if you have difficulty bending or reaching. What a doctor sees in the office is not always representative of how a patient functions each day. Be sure the form is completed accurately and truthfully.

An employer's long-term disability plan might have a much shorter payment period for mental illness than for other conditions. Pay special attention to this.

Some employer disability plans severely limit the length of time they will pay for a disability caused or contributed to by mental illness, compared to physical illnesses. Be especially mindful of the term, "or contributed by." The term leaves a grey area for disability reviewers to latch on to, and they might use that against you. Usually there are restrictions for alcoholism and drug abuse, as well. My employer would pay for a disability caused by mental illness for only two years. There may also be pre-existing condition limitations and other plan limitations.

To my knowledge, mental health parity laws still do not pertain to long-term disability plans.[50] You might not be familiar with parity laws. Parity, in terms of mental illness, requires insurers whose health plan offers mental illness benefits to provide the same level of benefit for mental illness as for other physical disorders and diseases.[51] Such benefits can include deductibles, copays, coinsurances, out-of-pocket limits, visit limits, and lifetime maximums.[52] Parity laws are complex and vary by state. Much depends on the number of employees an employer has, and other factors. I think that long-term disability plans that pay mental illness benefits differently from the benefits for physical disorders are unfair. If you are concerned about a mental illness limitation on your long-term disability plan, consult an attorney.

If you are taking a psychiatric medication strictly for physical reasons, be sure you doctor clarifies that in your file. Otherwise, an insurance company might conclude the medication is for psychological reasons. For example, some physical conditions can benefit from an antidepressant medication, although no psychiatric disorder exists.

A few years ago, I had to get a MRI of my foot. I thought I would not be able to keep my foot still as required during the test, so I asked my doctor for a pill to make me less aware of my discomforts. My doctor and I both agreed the prescription was not for mental illness. It was merely to help me get through the test because my foot was so uncomfortable. A disability reviewer read those notes and implied that I had been on the medicine for emotional reasons. My doctor had to write the insurance company a letter emphasizing that I did not have a mental disorder. The insurance company might try to corner you in any way they can. Ask your doctors to be sure their notes specify why you are taking an antidepressant medicine. You don't want an insurance carrier to unjustly limit your benefits.

The definition of disability can vary. Typically, long-term plans will consider you totally disabled if you cannot perform the duties of your own occupation for a certain period of time (usually twenty-four months), but thereafter, only if you cannot perform the duties of any gainful occupation. Other plans will consider you totally disabled only if you cannot perform the duties of any gainful occupation. State laws may vary. Waiting periods for disability also vary from plan to plan. Some plans might offer a cost-of-living increase, which is a great benefit.

Some employers will not allow you to make contributions to their 401k plans once you are receiving long-term disability benefits. Employers do not want to make long-term disability enticing. There may also be laws around this issue; consult an attorney for more information.

There will most likely be paperwork for tax withholding. Discuss it with your employer and tax advisor.

When applying for Social Security Disability Insurance (SSDI), hire an attorney, if you can afford one.

It's best to hire an attorney to help you apply for SSDI. If you can't afford an attorney, still apply if you think you deserve SSDI. You will be given forms to complete. If you are able, complete the forms yourself rather than having a Social Security employee fill out the forms for you. This will ensure that the forms are thoroughly completed; otherwise, an employee might misinterpret what you said or not state the details of your answers to the questions. If you are fortunate to have an attorney, discuss the forms with him or her.

Once you are on long-term disability, some employers will require that you apply for SSDI. They want you to also receive Social Security disability benefits so that some of their own costs will be offset. Your eligibility for SSDI is based on many factors. You also must have a certain number of work credits prior to your disability. Credits are based on earnings.

The following is a very simplified example of how an employer disability and Social Security disability plan might coordinate payments. Assume that you have a long-term disability plan for which your employer will pay you 50 percent of your basic monthly earnings. (Keep in mind, though, that most employers have a maximum amount they will pay an employee for the monthly disability benefit. You could get less than 50 percent if you have high earnings.) Let's assume, for this example, that 50 percent of your basic monthly earnings would give you $3,000 a month in long-term disability benefits. If SSDI also accepts you as totally disabled under its program, it will tell you how much you will receive from it. Assume, in this example, that SSDI gives you $2,000 a month. Some employer plans will offset the $2,000 and only pay you $1,000 a month for the long-term disability benefit. Various factors might be used to offset an employee's monthly benefit.

Plans vary. Ask your employer how it coordinates its disability benefit payments. If you need further information, consult with an attorney.

My employer wanted to enhance my chances of being approved for SSDI, so my employer paid the cost of an attorney. If your employer does not pay the costs for an attorney, call attorneys to compare fees.

Some lawyers will come to your house if you are unable to drive or travel. Your attorney will request notes from your doctors. Your attorney might ask that you obtain a letter from your physicians stating the nature and extent of your disability and your limitations. Get your doctor to include key points that Social Security wants addressed. It's important that your limitations are fully addressed, not just the diagnosis. It is imperative that the letter be truthful.

Once you are on SSDI for a continuous twenty-four months, you will usually automatically receive Medicare Part A. You will also be entitled to Part B, but will probably have to pay a premium for it. Contact the Medicare office for specifics pertaining to your situation. Parts A and B are offered earlier than twenty-four months if you are disabled by Lou Gehrig's disease.[53]

Your employer might require that you also have Medicare Part B in order to receive payment under its employer health plan. Employers want to offset their medical insurance costs, and Medicare sometimes pays medical claims prior to your employer plan. That results in less cost for the employer for your medical expenses. For several years, my employer paid the Medicare Part B premiums for me. Eventually those costs were turned over to me. Which carrier pays first depends upon various factors. Consult with your employer and Medicare to determine which carrier pays first for your situation.

Medicare is a government-sponsored program for those on SSDI and those aged sixty-five and older. For those on SSDI, Part A considers the cost of hospice care, home health or skilled nursing facility services, inpatient hospital services, and other inpatient services.[54] Part B considers the costs of outpatient care, including physician services, ambulance services, various screening tests, physical therapy, and other services.[55] For a complete list of coverages for Part A and Part B, contact the Medicare office.

Several years after my attorney completed my disability case, his office asked me if I wanted copies of my physicians' notes. When my attorney initiated my case, he had requested notes from all of my doctors. I told my attorney I wanted copies of all of the notes even though there was a small fee to receive them. It's good to have all of the notes in case something comes up for which you need that history. You may already have many of the notes if you previously requested them from your doctors. It's helpful to also request the notes from your attorney to be sure you have records of everything.

If you are totally disabled and have serious financial limitations, also ask your attorney or the Social Security office about the Supplemental Security Income (SSI) program, which is based on financial need.

The information given in the disability section of this book is based on the assumption that Medicare and SSDI are still in effect and that the programs have not changed. Government programs are subject to discontinuation.

Keep in mind that investigators may ask neighbors and friends their observations of your daily activities.

If you are on disability, friends, family members, and neighbors might be contacted by a disability reviewer. The reviewer might ask them what activities they have noticed you doing. For example, they may want to know if neighbors have seen you shoveling snow, mowing the lawn, or raking leaves. The disability reviewers want to be sure you are being honest in what you are telling the reviewer that you can and cannot do. If you have an invisible disability, however, this can be problematic. You may be perceived by others as being fine, when you are really not. Someone with an invisible impairment may even have been outside when they were not feeling good, but a neighbor looking at them could not see the pain they were in. A woman with multiple sclerosis told me that her neighbor did not understand the severity of her symptoms. Her neighbor had seen her in her yard during the moments she was feeling okay, and the neighbor made the assumption that she was completely better.

Years ago, I parked my car in a handicapped parking space to go to a urology appointment. My handicapped parking permit was hanging in the proper place in my vehicle. When I stepped out of my car, my foot was bothering me, the pressure in my bladder was intense, and I had tremendous fatigue from the chemotherapy I had received not too long ago. Someone looking at me, however, could not see my discomfort. After I walked a few yards, a woman came up to me and yelled at me for using the handicapped space. She said I looked too young to need a handicapped parking space and told me I did not look disabled. I politely told her that I did have problems. She screamed at me and then hastily walked away.

Another situation in which I could have easily have been misjudged was when I tried to shovel a very small amount of snow from my driveway. Because of a bad back, I had not shoveled snow for years. One morning, I noticed a very thin layer of snow upon my driveway. I pushed the snow across my driveway with a broom. I thought if I practiced doing a small amount during each storm that eventually I would be able to shovel more. All I did was push the broom once across my driveway. That was enough to flare my back up for days. I iced my back the entire day, on and off. Anyone driving by my house while I was using the broom could have assumed that I was going to do the entire driveway. They never would have known that just a few minutes later, I was inside icing my back.

You certainly don't want to hide out in your house to avoid nasty comments. You need to be aware, though, that others may be watching you and jumping to conclusions. Keep a daily log of all your symptoms. It can be helpful if you have to defend yourself in such scenarios for disability or insurance purposes. A friend of mine had a life insurance examiner follow her around. She called the insurance office to tell an agent she knew she was being followed and that she had invisible conditions.

Be aware that employer rehabilitation programs to facilitate a return to work may be different from a SSDI rehabilitation program.

At some point during your disability, your employer or doctor may suggest that you participate in a rehabilitation program. You may be on an employer disability plan, as well as SSDI. They may both have rehabilitation programs to encourage you to return to work. These different rehabilitation programs might have conflicting guidelines. They are distinct and operate somewhat independently. For example, an employer plan may give you a shorter trial-work period than SSDI's trial-work program. Also, an employer plan may use different assessment tools to judge your ability to return do work, regarding monthly income or work activities. Consult a lawyer for this situation, as you want to be sure you are following everything legally.

You might suddenly get a call from your employer's rehabilitation specialist. Mine called me just a few hours before she came to my house. I was disappointed that my employer sent someone over that didn't have much knowledge of my bladder disease. If the rehabilitation specialist didn't understand the ramifications of my disease, how would she adequately assess whether a rehabilitation program was suitable for me?

The process of applying for disability can be mind-boggling, but if you deserve the benefits, it's worth it.

Keep a History

Keep notes about your daily activities and limitations.

If you are on disability, keep a daily log of your symptoms and activities, if you can. Also keep a log of conversations you had with your practitioners. Write down the names of the people you spoke to, the department they work in, and the time of day you talked to them. You can refer to the log when you get your doctors' notes and confirm that the notes covered all aspects of your visit. Keep records of all phone conversations with claim representatives, nurses, lawyers, friends, family members, and anyone with whom you discussed your medical condition with. You might be surprised how valuable this history can be later on. A detailed history is especially helpful for disability reports and insurance appeals. Even if you are not on disability, your notes may come in handy for something unexpected in the future. Also keep track of your gas mileage to medical appointments in case you need that information for tax purposes. Don't count the mileage if you were using the transportation services and vehicles of others.

Keep a copy of your expired medical insurance identification card(s). They could come in handy for issues that may arise in the future.

Interacting with Attorneys

Thoroughly read all forms before you sign them. Check all forms for accuracy.

Don't let yourself be intimidated by attorneys. Discuss fees upfront, and be sure they are clarified. Copies, phone calls, e-mails, and faxes can add to the overall fee. If your case was originally scheduled for court, but ultimately settles out of court, ask your attorney if you will be charged additional fees if court proceedings were already initiated. Be sure your lawyer informs you of any settlement offers as they arise. Ask your attorney how long he or she thinks your case will take. Legal matters often take much longer to finalize than people realize.

Some people told me that their attorneys spent too much time going over what was discussed at a prior meeting. Don't expect an attorney to remember every detail of your prior visit. If your attorney spends an excessive amount of time going over items you had both previously discussed, however, it can be frustrating and waste a lot of a client's money.

When my husband and I looked over our wills that were drawn up by an attorney, we found numerous clerical errors. My husband and I arrived one hour early at our attorney's office to review our wills before we signed them. We did this because we anticipated there would be errors. There were many substantial errors, which took the office approximately an hour to correct.

Emotions

Caught in the Middle

Be assertive to meet your needs as well as the needs of disability reviewers, physicians, and your attorney.

If you are on disability, it can be frustrating to follow the correct protocol for your doctors, your attorney, and the disability reviewers, as well. They each have their own needs. In my situation, I knew my doctors' office notes had to accurately reflect what was discussed during the visits with my doctors. I also knew that the fine detail of what I was describing to my doctors would be important to disability reviewers. Some doctors asked me why I kept repeating the same thing at various visits. I did it so the notes would accurately reflect that I still had the same symptoms. I was disappointed when my doctor's notes indicated that a particular treatment did not help me, when I had clearly said it did. If something is alleviating your pain, you want the people reviewing your case to see that you were honest about it. The majority of my physicians' notes lacked the detail needed for disability reviewers.

If you are on disability, you might end up getting many more tests than you normally would, because you and the doctors are trying to find evidence to show the disability reviewers. A patient may then be perceived as anxious and compulsive for getting so many tests. If patients on disability don't undergo the tests suggested by their doctors, the patients might be judged as not following through on their doctor's instructions or as not trying to get better.

You might feel pressured to try treatments that you don't think will benefit you. If you turn down too many treatments, it can be viewed as if you are not trying to get better.

My attorneys had their own kind of detail and information that they needed. They wanted to receive letters from my doctors within a certain timeframe. Some of my practitioners were not able to deliver the letters on a timely basis.

The expectations of all parties conflicted, and it did not work in my favor. You have to be a good coordinator and manager to keep yourself afloat as a patient. You must be a proactive and persistent patient, despite resistance from others.

Patients Have Reputations Too

Tell your doctors if you think they are misjudging you.

Patients, not just doctors, have a reputation to uphold. It seems unfair that a patient's reputation can suffer because of clerical errors, a doctor's poor listening skills, and incorrect physician notes. I want my doctors to know I have taken into account all that they have said. I want them to remember that I have tried various medical treatments and that I'm trying to get well. I have often been misjudged because there was not enough time during an office visit for a thorough conversation. A doctor's hasty assessment of patients can unfortunately cost patients their reputation which results in patients not being believed or trusted. If you sense that you doctor is misjudging you, discuss it with your doctor. When I stood up for myself, some of my doctors were very willing to hear me out.

Many years ago, I went to an acupuncturist. My insurance carrier required that I get pre-approval for it to consider paying part of the acupuncture treatments. I asked my acupuncturist if he would write a letter to the insurance carrier. He wrote one, but said that I was being overly concerned about insurance. He said that none of his other patients ever requested him to write a letter. I was merely doing what my insurance company required.

Another doctor had suggested that I get several tests done. I had the tests, but I had previously told him that I did not think the tests were necessary. At my next appointment, he wanted to know why I had so many tests done. I spoke up that time, and he apologized. He actually is one of my favorite doctors, so I tried to be very tactful when I defended myself. It's critical for patients to speak up to protect their own reputations. If I hadn't spoken up, my doctor might have perceived me as an overly concerned patient. His notes might have indicated that I asked for too many tests. Those misperceptions could influence a disability reviewer's assessment of me.

If you are perceived as whiny or needy, your doctor may not take your medical complaints seriously. Such misperceptions can result in a doctor not initiating appropriate tests or failing to make an accurate diagnosis.

Take Care of Your Emotions

If you seek a counselor to help you deal with the emotional aspects of living with your chronic medical condition, look for one who specializes in chronic illness.

Being sick is tough. You might feel you don't deserve to be sick. Unfortunately, no matter how good a life you've led, you may still get sick. Allow yourself sad times if you experience them. It's natural to feel down when you can't do all the things you used to do. Celebrate your accomplishments, even if they seem small. I remember the thrill I felt simply being able to walk to the end of my block.

It can be helpful to get counseling to cope with the ups and downs of living with a chronic illness. Find a counselor who specializes in chronic illness or who is at least familiar with some of the distinct issues that illness brings. There are many feelings and concerns unique to those with chronic illness. For example, you may feel less bonded with family and friends who do not understand why you can't do the things you used to do. Others may expect you to snap out of your illness. You may also have financial and legal concerns. There's a great need for more counselors who specialize in chronic illness.

A counselor or doctor may know of support groups in your area that you can attend. Support groups can be comforting because members can share concerns and solutions related to the same condition you have.

Some people benefit greatly when a spiritual aspect is added to their counseling session. Pastors can be of great help. I think all counselors should be willing to incorporate some aspect of spirituality for their clients who desire it.

Don't give up on making yourself look and feel attractive.

Feeling physically attractive can boost your spirits. Getting a haircut or wearing a new outfit can be uplifting. It takes no more time to put on nice-looking clothes than it takes to put on sloppy ones. Don't fall into the trap of not taking care of yourself because you are housebound.

If you go out looking good, others may not realize the suffering you go through. They may discount your illness, thinking that if you look good, you must feel good. Dress nicely for yourself anyway. Those times of feeling good, even if temporary, can bring you the greatest joy.

The only time when you have to be careful not to look too good, if you are on disability, is at your doctor's office. If you look too good, a doctor might perceive you as being better than you are.

Since we're talking about looking good and feeling good, I thought I'd toss in a little tip about eyeglasses. When I was undergoing chemotherapy, I needed a new pair of glasses. I bought a beautiful frame that I loved. What I failed to realize was that when my hair grew in, those frames would look very different on me than they did when I wore a turban. Well, they didn't look so great after my hair grew in, so I ended up needing to buy another pair of frames. If you need glasses while you have temporary hair loss, try frames on while wearing a wig with a cut similar to your usual hair style. You will get a better idea as to what they may look like when your hair grows back. If you can afford it, you may want to buy a pair of glasses for when you are undergoing chemotherapy and another pair when your hair grows back.

If you have lost your hair because of a medical condition, perhaps you are considering wearing a wig. I got many for free at a local cancer facility. The person there told me not to try to duplicate my original hair style. I was told that a wig in a different style would appear more real to others. I found it to be true, so I opted for a wig with a short hair length. Try on different wigs to see what works for you. Some are much better quality than others. I ended up wearing a turban in the summer months and a wig in the cooler weather. You can even ask a seamstress to make a turban for you. Others prefer to go bald, and some people actually look quite attractive without hair.

Do Others Decide What Bothers You the Most?

Be honest with others as to what type of support you need.

You may have several ailments, but one that causes you the most trouble. Friends and family, however, may offer more support for a specific ailment they believe is the most important. It could also be that some people offer support for only those diseases they recognize, believe, or understand. When I was diagnosed with ovarian cancer, I was offered money and a lot of support, which I deeply appreciated. Yet I kept thinking how much more I needed that kind of support for my other problems. It then became apparent to me that others probably did not realize how difficult the other problems were for me.

I don't mean to discount my cancer by any means, but I knew once I had the hysterectomy and chemotherapy, I would probably be okay, based on what my doctor told me. My prognosis was excellent. Meanwhile, I'd have to live with other ailments for a much longer time. I have great respect for those with cancer and other diseases who must undergo multiple treatments. It takes tremendous courage and determination to battle the effects of chemotherapy, radiation, and other aggressive regimens.

Suppose a friend offers you $500 toward a certain treatment you are receiving. You may not need it for that purpose if your insurance is paying the full cost. If you also have another ailment, that costs you a lot each month, you could tell your friend that the money will be very helpful for that condition instead. This situation could be awkward, depending upon the relationship you have with the other person. On the other hand, if that person truly wants to help you, he or she may be very happy to help you in any way.

Two Friends Sick at the Same Time

Be respectful of each other's situation and needs.

It can be very challenging when two friends or family members are sick at the same time, since both need recognition and support. It can land them in an awkward situation in which they end up competing for each other's attention. Although both will want to help each other out, they also need to take care of themselves. If you are in this situation, share your concerns with the other person, and let him or her know how much you care. Be honest with each other about how much of a supporter's role you can offer. Neither of you will benefit if you try to take on more than you can handle.

Don't compare your pain to your friend's pain. You might think you are suffering more than your friend and feel a little jealous because you think that the other person doesn't have as much pain as you. Comparing pain is not a good thing to do and will most likely strain the friendship. Everyone handles pain differently. Respect each other in this way.

It may be that your friend is fine but has other family members who also need his or her time and attention. Be respectful of others by not being overly demanding for help.

People Who Tell You What You Can Do

When others doubt you, stand up for yourself.

Have others told you they don't understand why you can't do certain activities? They may tell you that they know others who have worse conditions than yours but that those people can still do certain activities. People with different, similar, or even the same conditions should not be expected to be able to perform the same activities. Each person is unique in limitations and how illness affects him or her. Be assertive in such situations, and stand up for yourself. Keep your cool and be tactful. People either believe you, or they don't, and there is not much you can do about it.

When people question me, I get really sad inside. I have had people tell me they do not understand why I can't swim, bike ride, or use a mobility scooter. I had several foot neuroma surgeries that resulted in my having very uncomfortable sensations in my feet. No matter what the activity is, my foot pulls and tugs and often prevents me from carrying out the activity.

One person told me her relative has only one leg, yet he can do most activities. She said if he could do it, I should be able to. She became rather angry when I explained that his situation was not mine. I feel a deep empathy for all patients who have to deal with such reactions from people.

Fear

Don't let fear stand in the way of your health.

Fear can get in the way of your making good decisions. Some fear is purposeful; yet if your mind goes into a state of panic about certain procedures, tests, or surgeries that may be good for you, fear can be counterproductive.

I was afraid to get a dental implant. I had been through so many medical and dental procedures over the prior twenty years that the thought of another procedure set me into a psychic spin. It was complicated by the fact that I had several opinions from different dentists. Many of their opinions and interpretations of an x-ray conflicted. At the end of it all, the implant was not a big deal, and the discomfort was minimal. I experienced all that fear for nothing.

I don't think any of my dentists truly understood the sheer panic I was in, having gone through so many medical and dental procedures in the past. I didn't emotionally feel like I could take on anything else. I made vague remarks about it, but I should have told them how bad my fear was, so we could have discussed ways to reduce my fears.

Some practitioners may not realize the extent of your fear. You may have been traumatized from a past treatment. Tell your practitioners if you think your fear is going to interfere with your treatment.

Special Diets and Social Situations

Inform your host of your food restrictions.

Many patients must follow a special diet. I've tried numerous diets over the years to see if they would alleviate my symptoms of interstitial cystitis. The diets have included yeast-free, gluten-free, sugar-free, and others. It can be difficult to stick to diets when you have social gatherings to attend. You may feel that you are being rude if you tell hosts that you are not able to eat certain foods they are preparing. It's tempting to cheat to make it easier for everyone. It's a shame to cheat, though, just to make others happy.

Discuss the problem with the host prior to the event. Some people will be very accommodating. You can suggest that you bring your own food if it's already prepared and simple.

I am surprised that some hosts don't take diabetes or high-blood pressure diets seriously for their guests. The wrong diet can send such people into life-threatening situations.

Be very tactful and polite when discussing your needs. A host might understandably be disappointed if you can't eat what he or she is planning to serve.

Participate socially in ways that you can.

Another social problem that can develop is that you may have the time, money, and energy to partake in only a limited amount of activities. Some people are at their best early in the morning and become fatigued by the afternoon. Many social activities take place in the late afternoon or early evening. This situation is a problem for those who need to wind down and rest at that time. Traveling far may result in having to stay overnight, if you are too fatigued to travel home. Such trips can get costly.

Don't let your limitations prevent you from attending some social events, even though you may not be able to fully participate. If you get fatigued, you can leave early, or ask the host if there is a place you can rest for a while. I usually opt to attend something for an hour or two and then leave. Know your limitations and work around them. Those who are truly housebound may benefit from communicating with others via computers or other remote devices.

I am not going to deny that some hosts might feel hurt or disappointed if you leave early. Years ago, if hosts were upset with me for wanting to leave early, I would stay to make them happy. That choice was not a healthy for me, and I physically suffered the consequences. Despite taking all necessary precautions, you might find that some events are best avoided.

Don't Assume Someone Is Strange

Don't be quick to judge others.

Do you have medical needs for which you need to carry around equipment or do something a bit unusual? An acquaintance of mine used to be a sales clerk in a department store. She frequently saw a customer sitting on a small cane chair in the store, and she thought it was very odd of the woman to do that. Decades later, when she saw me carrying a small cane chair to rest on, she realized the woman probably had also sat in the store for medical reasons.

On days that I cannot drive, I carry items that I need in a tote bag. I always have a small blanket in the bag. I need the blanket to sit on in my drivers' cars, because the dip in most car seats causes my back to hurt. The blanket fills in the dip perfectly. I also carry food, because I frequently get hungry because of my hypoglycemia. My tote does not have a zipper, so many of the items are visible to people passing by. One of my practitioners politely told me that I would no longer be able to use the bathroom in the building next to hers. The owners were locking it because a homeless person was going in there. We suddenly realized that they thought I was the homeless person. I had used that bathroom when I arrived early for a visit and when my practitioner's own bathroom was not available.

On another day, outside that same facility, a woman came up to me and asked me if I needed help. I was sitting on the steps because I was early for my appointment. I could not figure out why she was asking me if I needed help. It then dawned upon me that she probably saw the blanket and thought I was homeless. Even though I didn't need her help, I appreciated that she had respect and understanding for those in need.

On the few occasions that I went to a mall, my husband pushed me in a wheelchair. I needed the wheelchair only for distance. I could get in and out of it and then walk short distances in the stores. One day he wheeled me in front of a store, and then I got out of the wheelchair and walked around. A group of young girls started laughing and pointing to me. I heard one girl laughing about how it was strange that I could suddenly walk. She must have thought that all people in wheelchairs cannot walk at all, or perhaps she thought it was some kind of miracle that I could suddenly get up and walk!

I have only one brand of shoes that are comfortable for my feet. Because of problems from foot surgeries, I have not been able to tolerate any other shoes. The shoes are not stylish, which limits the type of outfits I wear. The shoes look hideous with a dress or skirt. Sometimes I dare to wear the shoes with a dress, anyway. At least my feet are as comfortable as they can be.

It's best not to make quick judgments about others.

Life after Appointments

Keep a social life besides your doctor appointments.

If you have a chronic illness and have been visiting your doctor's office for many years, you may get very comfortable over time with the office staff. If you have lost some of your friends because they did not understand your illness, it's easy to get too dependent on the various staff members. Paid employees can lend significant support, but should not be expected to fulfill your social needs. It is imperative to keep some type of social life aside from your medical appointments.

Please Believe Me!

Don't let others verbally abuse you or make you feel guilty if they don't understand your limitations.

One of the biggest obstacles for patients is doctors not believing their patients' symptoms and limitations, which results in patients spending time during office visits defending themselves. It's very unfortunate for patients to have to deal with that situation, and it puts a tremendous financial strain on our health-care system when time could be better spent helping patients. Friends and family members may not believe you either. You may be labeled as lazy, sickly, or craving too much attention. It's frustrating to be confronted with such disbelief.

In 1993 I went to a doctor because I had foot weakness. My doctor asked me to stand on my left foot. I had trouble balancing and could not stand on it without wobbling. The office notes said that the doctor was not sure if I could not stand or if I just thought I could not. I was shocked when I read those notes. The reason I went to the doctor was because of the foot weakness and heaviness in the foot. Why would I pretend not to be able to stand on it? If the doctor had believed me, it would have helped set me in the right direction sooner, in terms of treatment.

Another doctor told me that I could not have had cancer if I was still alive. He said the type of cancer I had was too aggressive and that no one could have lived through it. I found his comment insulting. I had several biopsies, and all the reports indicated cancer. Cancer was also found during the surgery. I also had one of the top cancer surgeons in the United States. I could not believe that I was being questioned about my cancer, simply because I survived.

If a person has a temporary impairment or is in the hospital, I think most people are very helpful and empathetic. I know people who have been suffering with an ailment at home, who receive little support from others; yet when they were placed in the hospital for testing, they suddenly received a lot of support. It seems that being in a hospital has something to do with how seriously people take your situation.

When a person has a chronic problem, getting support from others can get complicated. Those close to you may think you are exaggerating, especially if you have multiple ailments. One day I went into the supermarket and was able to get a few groceries. I had to leave earlier than I had intended, though, because of the intense fatigue in my feet and legs. I barely made it to the car. I sat there in tears, as I realized that others did not believe or understand my situation. Negative reactions I'd received from others over the years flooded my mind. I had been an active person, and it never dawned upon me that others might not believe the severity of my symptoms.

Sometimes you have to tell people what you can and cannot do, even if you know it might backfire. Some people won't want to listen to the whys. I think most people are supportive if you have a condition they are familiar with or if your test results reveal something concrete. If you fall into the category of invisible illnesses or don't have a diagnosis, then you might have a difficult time getting the understanding you deserve.

I often ponder why some people don't understand or believe others with certain medical conditions. Perhaps others are afraid of getting sick themselves. Also, we are a time-oriented society. People may feel your needs are too time consuming for them to deal with. It could be that some people have watched a television show in which celebrities or others were portrayed as being quite at ease with their condition. If you look behind the scenes, you will probably find that those celebrities also struggle each day. Some people may be jealous if you are not working and they are. Some people may think you are taking advantage of the disability system. There are various reasons why people dismiss others who have health conditions. Many people told me that negative reactions from others are one of the most difficult things that they deal with. The people that I know who have challenging medical conditions are some of the bravest and most determined individuals I've met.

Friends and family members may grow weary of a person talking over and over again about their medical condition(s). Most likely the person is seeking understanding, support, and for someone to believe them.

Several people I know with interstitial cystitis (IC) suffer each day. IC is a bladder condition that is not thought to be bacterial. One of the symptoms of IC is urinary frequency. In severe cases, frequency can be more than a hundred times a day. Most people with IC do not get a good night's rest because of nighttime frequency. I usually awaken several times each night. I've had nights that I have been up nearly twenty times, although more commonly I will get up four to six times. IC affects almost every aspect of life, including work life, sexual life, and social life. There is no cure for it, although treatments are available. Unfortunately, some people with IC do not have success with the available treatments.

Many with IC have told me that they feel that their friends and family members do not understand the difficulty they have. Some people have told me that their family members or friends suggested they wear diapers, but the solution is not so simple. Someone who urinates sixty times a day would need to carry around a lot of diapers, not to mention the expense of it. Wearing diapers daily could also lead to urinary tract infections and chronic irritations. Wearing a catheter all day could also lead to similar conditions or other problems.

IC is a difficult and lonely disease to live with. I know people with IC who chose to have their bladders removed. Removal of the bladder, however, can cause other serious problems. Some doctors and surgical team members don't understand the ramifications of IC. Some people with IC have told me their pregnant coworkers, who had to get up frequently during the night to urinate, got tremendous support from other coworkers. A person with IC, however, may have gotten up more than ten times a night and receive little support. There is a great need for public awareness of this disease.

People suffer from numerous conditions daily. Endometriosis is a very painful condition women can get that often goes undiagnosed. It's a chronic condition in which endometrial tissue like that in the uterus grows outside of the uterus. This displaced tissue grows into other structures and organs. Endometriosis can cause excessive vaginal bleeding and numerous other symptoms. My surgeon found endometriosis on my ovaries, rectal area, diaphragm, and liver. My endometriosis remained undiagnosed for nearly ten years. One of my prior neighbors told me that his ex-wife used to be in a lot of pain from endometriosis. He admitted to me that he always thought she was exaggerating her pain, which he said put a great strain on their marriage.

People with multiple sclerosis, mental illness, heart disease, autism, reflex sympathetic dystrophy, celiac disease, or lung disease, also have invisible symptoms. There are many more conditions that are also not easily noticed or given the recognition that they deserve.

"You Are Used to Being Sick"

If you feel you are being insulted, speak up.

An acquaintance of mine once came down with an illness. She was telling me how awful it was for her because she didn't know what it was like to be sick. She told me that it was easy for me when I feel bad, because I'm used to being sick. I understood her comment on an emotional level, since one has to get to a point of acceptance with one's illness; yet on a physical level, the fact that someone has pain often does not mean the person doesn't feel it just as much as someone who doesn't have it frequently. If you get hit in the head with a baseball bat once and more times later on, it's still going to hurt! Some people think they will never get sick or are not the type of person to get sick. If you receive insulting or misinformed comments from others, you need to stand up for yourself. Don't meekly accept rudeness from others. You obviously would not want to create a combative environment, but do politely defend yourself.

"Who Are You to Complain?"

Don't think that you always must be positive.

Some cancer survivors told me that some acquaintances criticized them if they complained about anything. They told them they should be happy they are alive and therefore should never complain again. Those standards are unrealistic for a person to meet for an entire lifetime. It's bad enough that those with cancer or other life-threatening illnesses had to go through what they did. It isn't fair that they should not be allowed to react as others do to normal situations and stresses in life. The fact that someone had cancer and recovered does not mean he or she won't have to vent once in a while.

Medical Terminology and Your Relationships

Sometimes it's best not to use medical terminology.

If you have a chronic illness and frequently see doctors, you will absorb a lot of medical terminology and knowledge. Before you know it, these terms become a normal part of your vocabulary. It's easy to start using medical terminology around friends and family members. They may become bored or irritated by it, though, as they won't know what you are talking about. They may also think you are trying to be some kind of hotshot or that you are odd.

Perhaps some patients hook up with each other and form friend-ships because they share an interest and medical vocabulary. They not only have someone they can relate to, but it's a safe place to talk without having to filter so much of their medical ter-minology. Keep a handle on using medical terms with others. Think back to when you were not sick. You don't want to dis-tance yourself from others. It's best not to bombard people with too many technical words.

Will You Be My Friend if I Can't Drive?

If you can't drive, let your friends know what transportation services you will be using, so they won't think you will be depending on them too much.

Some people told me that soon after they could no longer drive, several of their friends became more distant. Some of their friends even ended the relationship. Most likely the friends were afraid that the person would ask them for rides and impose on their time. If you can't drive anymore, openly and politely talk to your friends about it. If you will be using the services of public or pri-vate transit services, tell your friends and acquaintances. If your need for a ride from friends is only occasional, let them know. If your situation is temporary, tell them. Informed friends probably won't be concerned with your asking them for rides. Let them know all of the services that are available to you, if there are any in your area.

Silence Doesn't Mean They Don't Care

Be aware that everyone responds differently.

Don't assume that family members or friends don't care if they don't express their feelings to you while you are going through an illness. Some people have a hard time expressing themselves. They may be concerned that they might say the wrong thing and unintentionally hurt you. They might feel that words are just not adequate enough to express what they are feeling. If they are there for you and you can sense their support, don't get fixated on having them verbalize what they are feeling.

People Help in Different Ways

Appreciate the help you get.

Everyone has a different way of helping. Some people might offer to drive you to appointments, others to make you meals. Still others might offer to help you select a good doctor or medical facility. Some friends are most comfortable just listening to your concerns. Some people gave my husband and me money to go to nice restaurants and enjoy ourselves, because we had been through so much. Other family members and friends gave us money to pay bills. We deeply appreciated all of their help and kindness.

Each person has something unique to offer you. Don't expect one person to fulfill all of your needs.

Are You an Optimist, Realist, or Pessimist?

Don't buy into comments from people who imply your attitude caused your illness.

When a person has an illness, it's not uncommon for others to tell them to approach it optimistically. I have especially noticed this behavior toward people with cancer. Some patients have been given books on how to think positive, as if they can just snap out of their illness. Although the people who give such books mean well, it can be insulting to receivers. Such books can send a message that you got sick because of a pessimistic attitude. While a good attitude is helpful to have, many ailments have no correlation to attitude. How about babies born with medical conditions? Certainly the infants did not bring the medical condition upon themselves. Some people might argue that a mother's lifestyle and emotional state affect her genetic expressions, but more research is needed to validate that theory. I know many people who are enthusiastic, loving, good natured, and determined, who unfortunately still have a medical ailment to bear.

Each person has his or her own approach to dealing with illness. I have always considered myself to be a realist. When I first learned of my cancer diagnosis, I immediately faced all of the possible outcomes head-on. I read various books to learn what treatment options existed. I also called a cancer hotline and talked to other patients about their negative and positive experiences. After that, I allowed all my feelings to surface. I wanted to stare cancer in the face and not let fear bring me down. Once I began chemotherapy, however, I approached the situation entirely optimistically. That approach worked for me. I handle any obstacle that way. I like to be aware of all the bad and good of a situation, analyze how I can best handle it, and then move forward with a sense of optimism.

I have met other cancer patients who approached their cancer entirely optimistically from the beginning. They didn't want to talk to others about negative experiences. They considered only the treatment plan suggested by their doctor. This approach was suitable for them.

Some people appear pessimistic from the beginning of a diagnosis and throughout treatment which does not mean that they can't have a successful outcome. Continuous negativity, however, can drag a person down. You don't want a helpless attitude to cause you to give up on your treatments or not take care of yourself.

Sometimes others are too quick to label someone as a pessimist. Perhaps a person is having a difficult time processing all the feelings that go along with a medical diagnosis. He or she may just be temporarily releasing feelings of sadness and fear, which does not necessarily mean that the person is negative.

Each person has his or her own way of dealing with illness. People should not be telling others that the reason they are sick is that they brought it on themselves by a poor attitude. One could argue that certain health problems can be brought on by people not taking care of themselves. I don't deny that fact, yet numerous ailments are genetic or the result of our environment. Research will continue to reveal more about how important one's attitude is in staying healthy or recovering from an illness. It's important to have faith, hope, and perseverance; however, sometimes it's not fair that people get blamed for being sick.

Don't Lose Your Smile

Don't stop smiling just to please others.

After I spent years of having to be on the defense with medical practitioners and disability reviewers, it occurred to me that I was not smiling as much as I used to. I lost myself somewhere along the way. The constant battling with the claim offices, doctors, and disability reviewers was wearing on me. I also had been conditioned not to look too happy, lest someone not believe all the suffering I was going through. It took a lot of soul searching to get my smile back. Don't let the system smother your smile.

Have people asked you how you can smile when you have so many medical problems? When people ask me, their tone of voice determines how I react. Some have said it lovingly. Others have told me that I can't be in much pain if I can smile. Some of my limitations constantly bother me, but I've learned to smile anyway and be pleasant to others. I don't want to go around all day sad or angry at the world. I also have sporadic times when I do feel quite good, and then I am so happy that I'm not feeling awful at the moment, that I can't hide my smile. Why should anyone be penalized for smiling?

Do You Have So Many Medical Conditions That People Disregard Them?

Find less wordy ways to describe your illness to others.

You might have multiple medical ailments. If others hear you talking about all of them, it might overwhelm them. After a while, you might find them tuning out what you are saying. They may not believe that one person could have so many conditions at one time. Some people might believe you, but might categorize you as a person with medical issues, so they lose focus of the specific conditions that you have and do not realize how much you are suffering.

Fibromyalgia causes musculoskeletal pain in various areas of the body, and the symptoms can vary throughout the day. Those with fibromyalgia may suffer with back, neck, shoulder, hip, and foot pain all at the same time. Their discomfort might cause them to compensate in the way they handle their daily activities, which can result in even more pain and other problems. If your hip hurts, you might limp, which in turn might cause knee pain. When one part of the body is ailing, other parts of your body can suffer too.

I have fibromyalgia and have had times in which my foot problems flared up so much that I've had to use crutches for a few days to get around. Sometimes my foot problem can trigger another foot condition, such as tendonitis or plantar fasciitis. On some days the fibromyalgia results in my having to wear a neck brace.

Some people with fibromyalgia have told me that they feel that friends and family members with just one condition receive more support than they themselves get for their multiple symptoms. It can be frustrating to have various symptoms and feel that others don't understand the seriousness and limitations of each.

Others either don't realize what those with multiple symptoms go though, or perhaps others find it easier for themselves to lump multiple symptoms into one category. It's unfortunate when those who truly have many symptoms are dismissed by others who think they are exaggerating. Someone with one condition might be accepted more than a person who has that same condition and many more.

Instead of explaining each ailment to people, it's easier to say your condition causes pain in multiple areas of your body and that the symptoms vary daily. Very close friends, however, may be more tolerant of hearing more detail.

Do You Forget What Vacations Are Like?

Visualizations can recreate fond memories. If you can't physically travel, watch a DVD or something online that can momentarily transport you to a beautiful place.

Has it been a long time since you've had a vacation? One day, I realized I hadn't had a normal vacation in more than twenty years, so I closed my eyes and visualized many beautiful places I visited years ago. At first, my mind could not construct the images. Gradually, though, the images appeared, and I felt the greatest joy. I saw myself walking through the desert, running over sand dunes by an ocean, and strolling down a boardwalk. It felt so good to have those feelings and memories return, even if only in my mind.

If you are not able to take a long vacation, consider day trips. Even getting out for an hour or so locally can be uplifting. Often there are places close to home that you can explore and enjoy. Contact your state's tourism department to see if they offer free brochures on local events and places to go. Some libraries offer free passes to certain local attractions.

The Family Unit Needs Support

Be aware that others are affected by your illness too.

When one person in the family has an illness, it affects the entire family. It's also important to pay attention to what other family members are going through with their own illnesses. Sometimes counseling for the whole family can be helpful. Each family unit is unique, with individual needs. With certain diseases, tremendous time demands can fall upon a caretaker. The entire family needs to work together, and come up with a system that works for every-one in the family.

I get concerned when elderly grandparents, who have serious medical conditions, babysit for their grandchildren. Perhaps the grandparents' children do not understand the limitations that their parents' medical conditions present. Also, grandparents might be afraid to speak up about their difficulties. If grandparents have invisible impairments and do not share that information with their children, their children will not be aware of their parents' prob-lems. Some grandparents have told me they get fatigued when babysitting for extended times, but they don't want to tell their children. Certainly medical emergencies can arise with younger babysitters and even a child's parents; however, problems are most likely to occur with someone who knowingly has a serious or life-threatening medical condition.

I Used to Be Nice

Don't be so nice that you don't take care of your own needs.

You need to speak up and be persistent to get what you need as a patient. One of the most difficult things for me emotionally was that I had to transform my personality to get what I deserved at some medical offices. Some receptionists thought I was being too particular or making a big deal out of something. Although something might seem trivial to a receptionist or practitioner, it can be very significant for a patient. I learned to let go of worrying whether staff members liked me. I knew that if the staff was a bit irked by me that I was probably doing a good job of being a smart patient.

Gratitude

Give thanks for what you have.

With all the chaos that can surround you while attending to your health care, don't forget to be grateful for the good things you have. Give thanks to practitioners who support you and truly try their best to help you. Give thanks to your friends and family members who have stuck by you. Give thanks for moments of peace and quiet, although they may be few. If you believe in God or another higher power, give thanks for that presence too. Some may find it helpful to keep a gratitude journal.

Consider treating someone who has been very good to you, to breakfast, lunch, or dinner. If you are fortunate enough to have rides from friends and family members to your medical or dental treatments, consider buying each person a small gift and thank-you card to show your appreciation for their time and generosity. Put your creative mind to work and think of ways to thank others who have helped you out. If you are financially strapped, you can express your gratitude through a poem and give it to the person who helped you out. If you are getting rides from a service that you pay for, they usually will not allow their drivers to accept gifts. You can still verbally thank them and tell them how grateful you are for their services.

If a nurse, doctor, or staff worker has been very helpful to you, verbally thank them and let them know how much you appreciate their great service.

Good nurses should be applauded. Nurses work hard and can be your bridge to proper care. During my hospital stay for ovarian cancer, most of the nurses were very attentive to my needs. The nurses also lifted my spirit when I became weary.

Don't lose sight of those that truly do their best to help you out.

Where Do We Go from Here?

Aren't My Eyes, Teeth, and Mind Part of My Body?

If you think that limitations for benefits are not fair, speak up.

It astonishes me that many insurance plans have such limited coverage for vision, dental, and psychological services. I think the future of medicine will move in the right direction in this regard. Parity laws are already making a dent. Furthermore, the Patient Protection and Affordable Care Act (PPACA) impacts dental and vision plans in terms of how plans are offered.[56] The regulations pertaining to mental health parity, PPACA, and HIPAA are complex.

Write to insurance companies and federal representatives to discourage unfair vision, dental, and mental health limitations.

If you have questions about parity, PPACA, or HIPAA contact the National Conference of State Legislatures, U.S. Department of Labor, or an attorney. You can also contact your state Department of Public Health for guidance.

Educate the Public

Encourage our educational system to teach people about invisible illnesses and the needs of those with other health conditions.

Some people with health problems might be afraid that they will be viewed as wanting pity if they speak up about their conditions. They fear they might be ostracized which would result in them becoming even lonelier. Too often, those with chronic problems are dismissed by society and made objects of gossip.

Those with adverse health conditions need to reach out as a group. Educating the public is critical and could start with the public school systems. I believe that those with health issues are not asking others to totally revamp their lives on their behalf, but rather just want and need people's understanding and acceptance. I am very weary of seeing those with chronic problems dismissed by others so quickly. Those with limitations should not have to act like certain activities don't bother them just to please others.

You also have to hope that professionals treating you understand the limitations of your condition. Even a simple thing like getting your teeth cleaned can get very complicated if you have certain medical conditions. I think most practitioners understand limitations when the impairment is visible; if it's not, they may not realize what someone is going through.

The public also needs to be educated about invisible illnesses. Numerous patients have shared with me their frustration about others not understanding their invisible symptoms. For instance, some news reporters take pictures of people who do not look impaired but who are using handicapped parking spaces. The news media then broadcasts those pictures on television. Some of the people portrayed might have an invisible walking impairment, and face unfair criticism.

Our world is full of both healthy people and those that have medical conditions. Those with physical problems are sometimes shut out from others. We need to make room for them in our society. Sometimes, those with physical ailments just need another way of doing something. The end result can be just as good; they just have another way of getting there.

People with medical conditions should demand more respect from others regarding their illness. They should not let others be verbally abusive to them or make them feel guilty about things they can't change or do. I know several brave people with medical conditions who are dismissed by others. Their friends and acquaintances sometimes think they are exaggerating or being needy when they verbalized that they have trouble performing a certain task. I have seen others roll their eyes at them. I have grown weary of such disrespect. The more that people with health conditions back off to avoid confrontations, the less they will be able to move forward in this regard. I am not advocating aggressive confrontation with others, but that those with health conditions should not stand meekly on the sidelines. You need to tactfully speak up, and get the respect that you are entitled to. Perseverance is required and it will take years, most likely, before we see true acceptance from our society in this regard. Healthy people need to understand that not all illnesses have cures. Others have told me that their friends don't understand why a doctor can't cure their ailment.

I also realize many people are supportive to those with medical issues. They deserve a standing ovation, and then some. I have a deep gratitude for those kind-hearted individuals who do their best to help someone in need.

Telemedicine

Consider the use of telecommunication.

Telemedicine uses electronic communication to provide health care at a distance. Videoconferencing, remote monitoring of vital signs, and transmitting of images are all considered part of telemedicine.[57] This can be especially useful to patients who cannot travel or who live in remote areas. Telemedicine gives these patients access to professional urban medical centers that they could not otherwise access.

Although we may value telemedicine, we must ensure that it offers quality service. Our society must be sure that insurance laws, liability laws, licensing laws, and other aspects of health care keep pace with telemedicine as it continues to expand.

The Wisdom of Our Elderly

Be grateful for the elderly and what they offer.

I have a deep respect for elderly people and value their wisdom. I have sometimes seen the elderly being treated like children at nursing facilities, physicians' offices, and hospitals. Elderly people have years of experience and so much knowledge that is often overlooked by others. Just because their bodies may be frail does not necessarily mean that their minds are as well.

I don't think that others intentionally talk down to the elderly. Rather, I think our society tends to treat a frail elderly person as if they can't make their own decisions, or don't know what is best for them. They deserve so much more respect than that. Their physical complaints may be dismissed too easily by others who assume that old people don't know what they are talking about.

I have a vision of our school systems getting children more involved with the elderly. Elderly people could come into the class-rooms to speak about what they have learned in life. Students could volunteer to buy groceries for the elderly who cannot get out. Others could visit someone who is alone. This would teach children to have respect for elderly citizens. It is my hope that this same respect would then be reflected in nursing homes, hos-pitals, physicians' offices, and neighborhoods. Our society also needs to learn the importance of being patient with others. An elderly person who is frail may require more time in many aspects of their care. Let's give the elderly the time and respect that they deserve.

A Good Attitude Is Necessary for Good Care

Encourage a good attitude.

Over the years, I've realized that many of the careless medical errors I have come across were due to a staff worker having a poor attitude. Someone with a good attitude is friendly, patient, eager to learn, and willing to admit mistakes. Staff members should not get upset at patients for asking questions that are important to their care.

I also hope that doctors will recognize the importance of having a receptionist with a good attitude and kind spirit. After all, the receptionist is usually the first person a patient will meet when arriving at the office.

An employee with a bad attitude may be more apt to be careless. That can steer patients' health care in the wrong direction. Nurses, physician assistants, receptionists, and clerical workers, are key players in a doctor's office.

Employer Work Schedules and Employee Health

Encourage employers to examine how overtime contributes to medical costs.

I think employers who demand that their employees work excessive overtime are increasing health costs in this country. Lack of sleep and stress contribute to chronic health conditions.

For instance, one summer, my former employer required some of its employees to work so much overtime that they didn't even have time to go to a dental or doctor appointment. Those employees rarely got to go home to a nice dinner and spend time with their families. They slept very few hours per night.

I once met an executive who held a very high position at an insurance company. He told me he made all of his employees leave on time. He wanted them to take care of their personal needs and to enjoy their families when they got home. He knew they would then be more productive. He also thought it would cut down on the employer's costs because employees could then take care of themselves. I wish more employers understood how smart his reasoning was.

Educate Doctors about Disability

Encourage medical schools to offer classes about the disability system.

Doctors need to be properly trained in handling disability paperwork. This training would help physicians understand how critical it is for them to keep detailed and accurate patient notes. Too often, doctors dismiss the importance of thorough notes. Physicians' notes have a lot to do with a patient's disability and life insurance determinations. Such notes can impact a chronically ill patient's future and financial health. There should be standardized guidelines for doctors to use when writing patient notes. Accurate notes are important whether a patient is on disability or not. Perhaps a special department could be established at state public health offices to enhance rules regarding office notes.

Do Residents Need More Sleep?

Encourage legislation that allows residents to get good sleep.

Lack of sleep among residents is another area that society needs to examine more closely. Haven't we all heard of residents having to work long hours with little sleep? On the one hand, perhaps this environment prepares medical residents for the real world when emergencies come up. Yet if residents are very tired, they are more prone to making errors. In July 2011, new standards were set that restrict the amount of hours residents can work, but sleep deprivation and long hours still exist.[58]

Trends

Keep informed.

The health industry is constantly changing. Some hospitals are creating their own insurance-like setups that bypass insurance companies.[59] Increasingly, doctors are leaving their own practices to become employed by hospitals.[60] Such trends will have an impact on how doctors deliver health care to their patients.

Patients have an increasing responsibility to manage their health. The focus of health care seems to be shifting to a preventive approach and keeping patients healthy.

New technology will enable more accurate diagnoses and improve surgical techniques. Already, robots are used for some surgical procedures. It may become common to use robots in nursing homes to get patients out of bed, pick up patients who fell, and deliver medication.[61] The use of robots in nursing homes will reduce costs and improve efficiency. Better methods of monitoring vital signs are continuously being developed. Bio-connectivity is a term used to describe technologies that connect patients at home to medical monitoring devices.[62] Some systems allow transmission of EKG's, blood pressure, and glucose levels.[63]

Research of personalized medicine is finally making some headway. [64] Fortunately, this may help change the attitudes of doctors who believe that all doses and types of medicine are appropriate for all adults.

Our society is experimenting with cars that drive themselves. Such technology is extremely advantageous to people who have physical limitations that currently prevent them from driving.

The concept of patient-centered medical homes offers a promising approach to deliver care. There is no standard definition of a patient-center medical home.[65] In theory, patient-centered medical homes emphasize improved doctor-patient relationships, team-based care, and prompt care; pilots of the homes are ongoing. [66] Although the aim of patient-centered medical homes is to improve health care, we must ensure that the homes do not succumb to bureaucratic pitfalls.

Health insurance carriers will more closely monitor claims to suggest effective treatments to manage patients' health care. Some insurers directly communicate with patients' physicians to take steps to improve the health of patients. My insurance carrier sent me a letter suggesting a specific medication to help my medical condition. My insurer also sent that information to my doctor. I think such involvement from an insurance carrier is intrusive; it's also disrespectful to doctors. Some insurers will use registered nurses to oversee the management of patients' with chronic conditions.[67]

Alternatives to nursing homes may become more common. Sidekick homes are small cottages designed for those with limited abilities that go in a homeowner's backyard.[68] Med Cottage is a small mobile home with many high-tech assistive features that you can place on your property.[69] Obviously, you have to be able to afford the units, but they may cost much less than care in a nursing home. A two car garage can be converted to an apartment to create a living area.[70]

Expect changes in how employers offer health benefits to their employees.

Expect to see more vending machines that dispense prescription drugs to authorized clients.

Traveling abroad for medical care is not uncommon as the cost of health care in the United States increases. This trend will probably continue as both individuals and insurers seek to lower health costs. You can explore accredited off-shore hospitals at www.jointcommissioninternational.org.[71]

New trends will continue to emerge. Keep informed so you do not lose touch with the latest advances in health care.

Conclusion

My hope is that doctors will not be so quick to label patients as having a psychological disorder when nothing shows up on tests. Perhaps no test has been developed to detect the patient's disorder. Medical research and technology progress each year, which gives society the hope that we will solve many of our medical mysteries.

Doctors should applaud patients who are brave enough to ask questions. Many people told me that their doctors dismissed them because they asked intelligent questions during an office visit. Inquisitive patients are sometimes regarded as difficult or compulsive. Such reactions from physicians are not only hurtful to their patient's care but also unethical. Your well-being, and sometimes your life, depends upon you watching out for yourself.

It is also my hope that practitioners will recognize the ramifications of clerical errors. Hospitals and medical institutions should hold classes for employees about the impact of clerical errors. Such errors severely affect patients and can even result in their death. Clerical errors are made by doctors, physician assistants, nurses, receptionists, other medical staff members, and even patients. All should be trained to be on the lookout for errors.

There is a great need to train doctors and staff members about pre-operative and post-operative care issues. I have had several surgeries in my lifetime, and after each, I was given only basic discharge instructions for my immediate care when I got home. No one informed me of the many other issues I might encounter over the next several weeks. It's helpful for patients to know what reactions after a surgery are normal and what reactions might be a good reason to call the doctor. I don't think physicians realize how much time and effort it takes for their patients to prepare for a surgery and after-care.

One of my former doctors, now deceased, told me that he felt terrible about how little time the insurance companies allowed him to examine his patients. I appreciated that he shared his thoughts with me, and I respected his honesty. Some doctors rudely rush me out of their office and quickly dismiss my issues. I'd rather have doctors that tell me I'm smart to ask questions, but that the insurance company is not allowing enough time for further discussions.

The health-care system in this country seems to be in a down-ward spiral. Few people may even want to become doctors if insurance company guidelines don't allow doctors to adequately treat patients. Friends have already told me that their doctors are retiring early because they don't like the constraints of our health-care system. Doctors might be frustrated by patients who are complaining that they are not getting the care they deserve. Many doctors have too much paperwork to allow them to give more time to their patients.

Patients and doctors both battle the constraints set by our health-care system. I hope that doctors and patients will unite to bring our health-care system to a higher standard.

It's important that patients and doctors develop a good working relationship. Seminars in which doctors and patients address each other's needs would be helpful. Physician assistants must be involved because they are taking over many aspects of patient care.

Certainly there are many fine doctors and medical professionals. Nurses, lab workers, physician assistants, and clerical staff have demanding jobs. I am thankful for all medical professionals who treat diseases and do their best to alleviate their patients' pain. It's hard to envision a society without doctors. We don't want to lose sight of the many professionals who are helping us; yet something is lacking in our health-care system. What's lacking is time for practitioners to adequately do their jobs.

As problems of our health-care system escalate, good attitudes are diminishing. Workers and patients are stressed from the inef-ficiency and ineffectiveness of our health-care system. Often, patients' concerns are dismissed and diagnoses made too quickly. Treatment plans that are life-altering for patients are sometimes made in office visits of fifteen minutes or less; hasty strategies are not always effective.

Some doctors have taken the Hippocratic oath that they will apply measures that benefit the health of their patients.[72] Yet, aren't patients being harmed by brief examinations and dismissal of their symptoms? Key executives of health insurance companies should be required to take an oath that their insurance regulations will not be such that they prevent doctors from delivering high-quality care to patients.

The relevance of the Hippocratic oath to modern society has been questioned, and over the years the oath has been rewritten into various versions to meet cultural demands.[73] As the oath continues to be modernized, may we never cease to uphold its ideals of ethical standards and to remind ourselves that the health of patients should be considered above all else.

About the Author

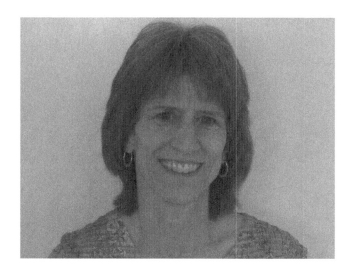

Patricia graduated *magna cum laude* from Central Connecticut State University with a bachelor of arts in psychology. She has worked in various jobs since 1970, including a medical benefits trainer position at a major insurance company. For several years, she volunteered as an assistant Connecticut state coordinator for the Interstitial Cystitis Association. She also formed and conducted a support group for those with interstitial cystitis. Patricia has initiated and participated in medical-related radio and television segments. She considers her most valuable experience, however, to be learning to live with the challenges of chronic illness.

Notes

Appointment Issues

[1] "About the Joint Commission," The Joint Commission, accessed September 22, 2011, http://www.jointcommission.org/.

[2] "What is Accreditation?," The Joint Commission, accessed February 6, 2012, http://www.jointcommission.org/.

[3] "Contact Us," American Board of Medical Specialties, accessed August 19, 2011, http://www.abms.org/.

[4] "Certification Matters: FAQs about Board Certification," American Board of Medical Specialties, accessed February 14, 2012, http://www.certificationmatters.org/faqs.aspx.

[5] Lisa Zamosky, "More Hit with Fees for Doctor's Extra Phone Calls, Filings," *Hartford Courant,* January 11, 2012, sec. D.

Inside the Office

[6] Lucas Mearian, "Hospital Turns to Palm Reading to ID Patients," *Computerworld,* June 16, 2011, 2.22 p.m. (EST), http://www.computerworld.com/.

[7] Emily Coakley, "Patient Palm Readers the Latest Effort to Digitize Health Records," *FindingDulcinea,* April 7, 2009, www.findingdulcinea.com/.

[8] Ibid.

[9] *Health Information Privacy,* U.S. Dep't of Health & Human Servs., http://www.hhs.gov/ocr/privacy/hipaa/understanding/summary/index.html (last visited May 24, 2012).

[10] Ibid.

The Waiting Room

[11] Richard Laliberte, "Where the Germs Are," *Woman's Day,* October 17, 2011, 89.

The Nurse Calls You In

[12] Alan L. Rubin, M.D., *High Blood Pressure for Dummies* (New York: Wiley, 2002), 17.

[13] Ibid., 18.

[14] Health Gear Inc., accessed September 21, 2011, http://www.healthgearweb.com/.

[15] Jimmy Biggerstaff, "Gowns Take a Little Thread, a Lot of Love," *Hi-Desert Star,* August 27, 2011, http://hidesertstar.com/news/article_b84f86e4-5035 -5013-b9d0-9d5786346bcd.html.

The Visit with Your Doctor

[16] "Independence at Home Act to Facilitate Aging at Home," Opinion, *Capecodonline,* June 6, 2011, http://www.capecodonline.com.

[17] Ibid.

After the Visit

[18] Phone conversation with State of Conn. investigations employee, anonymous per author (Sept. 14, 2011).

[19] *Practioner Complaints – Frequently Asked Questions,* State of Conn., Dep't of Public Health, http://www.ct.gov/dph/cwp/view .asp?a=3121&q=437134&dphNAV_GID=1821 (last updated Mar. 24, 2009).

[20] Phone conversation with State of Conn. investigations employee, anonymous per author (Sept. 14, 2011).

[21] David L. Blecker FACP, "Building Better Patient Notes by Using Templates," Archives, *ACPINTERNIST*, October 1998, http://www.acpinternist.org/.

[22] Ibid.

[23] Richard Knox, "Doctors Don't Agree on Letting Patients See Notes," morning edition, Your Health, *NPR*, September 21, 2009, http://www.npr.org /templates/story/story.php?storyId=112971637.

[24] Ibid.

[25] Tom Delbanco et al., "Open Notes: Doctors and Patients Signing On," *Annals of Internal Medicine* 153, no. 2 (July 20, 2010): 121, http://www.annals.org/content/153/2/121.full.

[26] Ibid., 122.

[27] *Understanding Health Information Privacy,* U.S. Dep't of Health & Human Servs., http://www.hhs.gov/ocr/privacy/hipaa/understanding/index.html (last visited May 24, 2012).

[28] Kelly Mclendon, "Electronic Records for All Patients Mandated by 2014," *Spacecoastmedicine*, August 3, 2009, http://www.spacecoastmedicine .com/2009/08/electronic-records-for-all-patients-mandated-by-2014.html.

[29] Shelley DuBois, "Electronic Medical Records: Great, but Not Very Private," Fortune, *CNNMoney.com,* October 6, 2010,11:15 a.m. (EST), http://money .cnn.com/.

[30] Ibid.

Prescriptions and Tests

[31] Joanne Chen, "Don't Get Surgery in July," *Prevention,* July 2011, 107.

[32] Phone conversation with manufacturer representative, anonymous per author, August 24, 2011.

[33] Phone conversation with pharmacist, anonymous per author, August, 24, 2011.

[34] Phone conversation with pharmacist, anonymous per author, August 24, 2011.

[35] Tara Parker-Pope, "Keeping Score on How You Take Your Medicine," Health, the *New York Times* online, June 20, 2011, http://well.blogs.nytimes.com/2011/06/20/keeping-score-on-how-you-take-your-medicine/.

[36] Ibid.

[37] Mary Brophy Marcus, "The Physician Assistant Is in – Just Not in a Doctor's Office," *USA TODAY,* August 29, 2011, sec.B.

[38] Ibid.

The Consequences of Clerical Errors

[39] Katharine Greider, "Your Health," *AARP Bulletin,* March 2009, 13.

Surgeries, Surveys, Rooms

[40] William Weir, "Drug Shortages: Hospitals Forced to Scramble Daily," *Hartford Courant,* January 5, 2012, sec. A.

[41] Ibid., A11.

[42] Joanne Chen, "Don't Get Surgery in July," *Prevention,* July 2011, 103.

[43] *Are You a Hospital Inpatient or Outpatient?,* Centers for Medicare & Medicaid Servs., Publ'n 11435, http:www.medicare.gov/library/pdfnavigation/pdfinterim.asp?Language=English&Type=Pub&pubid=11435 (last updated Feb.17, 2011).

[44] Ibid.

[45] Ibid.

[46] William Weir, "Quest for Prevention," *Hartford Courant*, October 20, 2011, sec. B.

[47] Ibid.

[48] Joanne Chen, "Don't Get Surgery in July," *Prevention*, July 2011, 102.

[49] Josh Kovner, "Patients Didn't Get Meds," *Hartford Courant,* September 13, 2011, sec. A.

Disability and Attorneys

50 American Psychological Association, employee anonymous per author, e-mail message to author, January 20, 2012.

51 *State Laws Mandating or Regulating Mental Health Benefits,* National Conference of State Legislatures, NCSL Health Program, Denver, http://www.ncsl.org/default.aspx?tabid=14352 (last updated December, 2011).

52 Ibid.

53 *Sign Up for parts A & B, Medicare,* http:www.medicare.gov/navigation /medicare-basics/sign-up-part-a-and-part-b.aspx? (last visited Feb. 8, 2012).

54 U.S. Dept. of Health & Human Servs., Centers for Medicare & Medicaid Servs., *Medicare & You 2012,* 33-53 (Aug. 2011).

55 Ibid.

Where Do We Go from Here?

56 "Health Insurance Reform: What Does It Mean for Dental and Vision Plans," Benefit Mall, accessed December 5, 2011, http:// www.benefitmall.com/News-and-Events/Legislative-Updates/ Health-Insurance-Reform-What-Does-It-Mean-for-Dental-and-Vision-Plans/.

57 "Telemedicine Defined," American Telemedicine Association, accessed October 5, 2011, http://www.americantelemed.org/.

58 Michael Breus, PhD, "Sleep Well," *WebMD* (blog), http://blogs.webmd .com/.

59 Anna Wilde Mathews, "The Future of U.S. Health Care," *The Wall Street Journal* online, Health sec., December 12, 2011, http://online.wsj.com/article /SB10001424052970204319004577084553869990554.html.

60 Editor (Anonymous), "10 Healthcare IT Trends to Watch in 2010," *Healthcare Technology Online,"* January 14, 2010, http://www.healthcaretechnologyonline.com/doc .mvc/10-Healthcare-IT-Trends-To-Watch-In-2010-0001.

[61] John Stewart, "Ready for the Robot Revolution?" *BBC News,* Technology, http://www.bbc.co.uk/news/technology-15146053.

[62] "Biotechnology for Your Health, *HealthGrades Advisor,* http://www.healthgrades.com/cms/newsletters/hg-advisor.

[63] Ibid.

[64] William Weir, "Tackling Medicine's Next Frontier," *Hartford Courant*, May 29, 2012, sec. A.

[65] "Health Policy Brief," *HealthAffairs.org,* September 14, 2010, http://www.healthaffairs.org.

[66] Ibid.

[67] Matthew Sturdevant, "Cigna Adds Network to Care Initiative," *The Hartford Courant,* May 30, 2012, sec. A.

[68] Ryan, "Caregivers Cottages: Bringing your Loved Ones Home." *Caregiving.com* (blog), *August 27, 2010,* http://caregiving.com/2010/08 /caregiver-cottages-bringing-your-loved-ones-home/.

[69] Ibid.

[70] Ibid

[71] "Accreditation for Hospitals," The Joint Commission International, accessed May 26, 2012, www.jointcommissioninternational.org/.

Conclusion

[72] Peter Tyson, "The Hippocratic Oath Today," NOVA, http://www.pbs.org /wgbh/nova/body/hippocratic-oath-today.html.

[73] "Hippocratic Oath," *Absolute Astronomy*, accessed February 13, 2012, http://www.absoluteastronomy.com.

CPSIA information can be obtained at www.ICGtesting.com
Printed in the USA
LVOW011559291112

309390LV00014B/1259/P